Medicine without Meds

Transforming Patient Care with Digital Therapies

DEAN HO

YOANN SAPANEL

AGATA BLASIAK

JOHNS HOPKINS UNIVERSITY PRESS | *Baltimore*

© 2023 Johns Hopkins University Press
All rights reserved. Published 2023
Printed in the United States of America on acid-free paper
9 8 7 6 5 4 3 2 1

Johns Hopkins University Press
2715 North Charles Street
Baltimore, Maryland 21218
www.press.jhu.edu

Library of Congress Cataloging-in-Publication Data is available.

ISBN 978-1-4214-4703-2 (hardcover)
ISBN 978-1-4214-4704-9 (ebook)

A catalog record for this book is available from the British Library.

Special discounts are available for bulk purchases of this book. For more information, please contact Special Sales at specialsales@jh.edu.

CONTENTS

It Is Time for Health Care to Embrace Patients
D. A. Wallach

D. A. Wallach is a venture capitalist and health care innovator focused on technologies poised to reinvent medicine. Industry-defining companies backed by the funds he cofounded—Time BioVentures and Inevitable Ventures—have included Beam, Glympse, Doctor on Demand, Devoted Health, and Neuralink. Wallach is an acclaimed recording artist and active in the nonprofit space focused on preventive medicine and patient support.

THROUGH THE LENS OF A CONSUMER AND TECH INVESTOR
Early-stage tech is fascinating. As an investor, I follow related developments on both micro and macro levels: advising startups at the academic stage while observing global trends being shaped by (and shaping) consumer demands. While I started my investing journey in technology with companies including Spotify, SpaceX, and Ripple, over time I developed a keen interest in health care. Carrying over my understanding of the dynamics of innovation to this sector, I am impressed by how much room for improvement there is in terms of consumer experience. Health care is one of the last frontiers where this shift in focus is still just beginning.

Coming into the health care field from the perspective of an investor "trained" in consumer technology, I was, and still am, shocked by the limited role consumers—patients—play in driving the demand for new solutions and high-quality user experiences. Instead, innovation in this field is commonly stewarded by payer demands, even though in the health care systems of developed markets payers are typically not the patients, but private or public insurers. Their motivations and objectives, as well as those of other stakeholders, may not be aligned with the needs and desires of patients—the population that the system should aim to serve.

Beyond this misalignment of stakeholders, there is a general lack of impetus for change on the part of gatekeepers with an interest in maintaining the status quo. The traditional incentive system behind technology adoption—staying competitive—is inoperative in health care, which is dominated by decision-making processes between payers (insurers) and providers (hospitals and clinics) that are not well understood. For potential investors interested in the sector, this opacity translates into a reluctance to take on investment risk without having a clear vision of the systems' workings and reliable drivers of future returns. In short, investors are wisely skeptical of the potential for innovation alone to produce successful, rapidly scaling companies. Yet, without private funding much of the innovation potential simmering in early-stage health technology, startups cannot be realized, resulting in an abundance of great technologies that languish at the proof-of-concept or pilot stage.

But there are reasons to be hopeful. The COVID-19 pandemic that put the world on pause and pushed much of health care delivery outside the hospital and into people's homes may well turn out to be an inflection point that shifts the balance of power. Many of the digital solutions for remote patient monitoring, adherence to treatment, and disease self-management that emerged in the aftermath of this pandemic may be here to stay, and they hold the promise of finally empowering patients with the decision-making power they never quite had before.

BUILDING VENTURES TO REINVENT HEALTH CARE

Without a doubt, the increased openness to remote patient care solutions paired with unprecedented advances in digital technology will serve as catalysts for health care innovation. Putting patients at center stage requires a technological engine that personalizes care with treatments optimized to each patient according to their genetic and physiological profile, lifestyle, and needs. This space is ripe for new technologies that can monitor, diagnose, and treat an affected population without losing the granular level of focus on each individual patient.

The time is right for budding entrepreneurs in this space to get investors' attention and the support they need to turn their ideas into viable, scalable products. A successful digital health endeavor is a convergence of substance and sales. Substance means technology, team, operation, execution, business strategy, and timing. Sales means the entrepreneur's ability to convince investors, employees, buyers, and end users of the value and impact of their solution by sharing a vision that is too good to miss. Being successful at balancing these elements is a unique predisposition and a rare one to come across.

To build a venture, entrepreneurs must have strong self-awareness and team-building skills. They need to understand their shortcomings and be willing and able to address them by surrounding themselves with the right people. Thus, a founder who is a technical wizard would be wise to team up with an experienced business strategist and an effective communicator; one who is a physician by training may want to join forces with a user-experience researcher, a software developer, a marketer, or so on. The most innovative companies are those formed by groups of people with complementary skills.

WHAT'S NEXT?
Digital health has the potential to reinvent health care. Wider stakeholder acceptance notwithstanding, it is within the reach of digital health entrepreneurs to tip the scales and transform piecemeal digital health inventions into large-scale health care innovation that embraces patients. It takes audacity to try and wisdom to know what the process entails. But while audacity may come naturally to an entrepreneur, where can one find the wisdom? Reading this book is a good place to start.

Traditional health care has a new ally. Patients with sleep disorders, back pain, and diabetes are now being prescribed app-based treatment in place of a drug. Algorithms are helping cancer patients to manage their symptoms. Video games are improving the attention span of children diagnosed with ADHD.

A new class of medicine, called digital therapeutics (DTx), is gaining traction and transforming the way patients engage with the health care system. Yet, as a patient, you may have never heard of this burgeoning field.

In this book, we speak to innovation and business leaders from all corners of the health care universe who are involved in designing and building tomorrow's DTx. They include clinicians, researchers, engineers, patients, startup founders, and corporate executives. We share their insights on how DTx can deliver value beyond the technology, address the challenges of implementation in existing health care models, and propose a way forward by revolutionizing care delivery. Through a learning lens, we also take a look at DTx innovations to date and analyze the key factors for their successes as well as their failures.

It is time to realize the potential of DTx, and we are bringing all stakeholders along on this journey that will ultimately bring reimagined health care to all.

MEDICINE WITHOUT MEDS

The Context

You know that discomfort you feel in your lower back every once in a while? Or that sharp pain shooting down your leg when you stand up too quickly? You have probably experienced low back pain at some point in your life, which is similar to over 80% of the population.[1] How have you dealt with it? For 56-year-old Simon, a "slight discomfort" (as he described it) did not stop him from his daily activities at first, so he didn't really pay attention to it. Over the years, though, the pain became more present, persistent, and sharp—evolving from a dull ache to chronic pain. Eventually he even had to take time off from work. Walking the dog became difficult. Playing with his kids was a struggle. Lifting grocery bags was impossible.

Despite remarkable advances in medicine, a common health problem such as low back pain is still mainly treated with analgesics. Sadly, they are effective in relieving the symptoms but not the underlying cause, which often remains unknown and therefore unaddressed. To complicate matters, Simon doesn't remember when the pain started or what triggered it. He simply knows, as his doctor had repeatedly told him, that he should move more, lose some weight, and lead a more active lifestyle. But do we all always follow our doctor's advice?

Over the years, Simon has had many consultations—not only with his family doctor but also with chiropractors, physiotherapists, and pain therapists—in search of a remedy. Physical therapy, rehabilitation, spinal manipulation, you name it: Simon has tried them all and spent an inordinate amount of time and money doing so. Fortunately, Simon's doctor was able to suggest a new approach—a mobile app for chronic pain relief. Hopeful that it would help him take control of his pain, Simon did not hesitate, especially since the solution promised to take only 10 minutes a day.

A medical and technological novelty for Simon, the app uses virtual reality supported by the latest scientific evidence in digital training, pain education, and psychology to deliver a behavioral intervention that may work as well as, and maybe even better than, medication. Over the course of a few weeks, the app "nudged" Simon to take a comprehensive approach to managing his pain through:

- *Exercise*: tailored to alleviate his pain and keep his body active;
- *Relaxation*: mindfulness, breathing, and progressive muscle relaxation techniques; and
- *Knowledge*: general pain and back pain–specific education modules to control the perception of pain.

Guided by the app, Simon received this regimen that adjusted itself to match his progress. For instance, when the app detected his motivation waning, a dedicated coach "intervened" in an attempt to reenergize him through interactive question and answer sessions.

After three weeks of daily use, Simon began to notice improvements as he gradually learned how to take control of his pain. This motivated him to finally start making adjustments to his sedentary lifestyle and in four months, Simon was pain-free for the first time in 20 years. Today, he no longer needs his pain medication—what a relief! If life is better without painkillers, it is much better without any pain at all.

Low back pain is the leading cause of activity limitation and absenteeism from work, resulting in significant medical burden and economic cost.[2] Consequently, it has become a major global public health problem.[3] As the world population ages, the prevalence of low back pain is projected to increase substantially due to spinal deterioration of older people in ever greater numbers.

Fortunately, health-focused technology, such as the mobile app that helped Simon gain control over his back pain, offers hope to the 540 million individuals estimated to be experiencing low back pain at any one time.[4] These types of apps represent a new class of medicine called digital therapeutics (DTx). Like drugs, DTx have to fulfill stringent requirements that demonstrate their safety and efficacy through rigorous clinical trials before they can be prescribed (we will discuss this at length later in the book). But most importantly, beyond back pain, DTx are clinically useful for a broad spectrum of behavioral, mental, and physical diseases and disorders. As such, they are regulated as "software as a medical device."

While we chose to share Simon's story of dealing with low back pain, we could have also shared the stories of Sarah, Elena, or Jin and how they are dealing with high blood pressure, high blood glucose, hypertension, excess weight, or early signs of dementia. Globally, one in three adults live with more than one chronic condition, whereas in the United States alone up to 60% of Americans have one or more preventable chronic diseases.[5] Examples include:

- *Cardiovascular diseases*: the leading cause of death globally, taking an estimated 17.9 million lives each year.[6]
- *Diabetes*: the world's fastest growing chronic condition and already one of the most costly and burdensome chronic diseases.[7] One in 11 adults has diabetes and one in two adults with diabetes is undiagnosed.[8]
- *Cancer*: one in two people will be diagnosed with cancer in their lifetime.[9]
- *Dementia*: someone in the world develops dementia every three seconds, adding up to nearly 10 million new cases every year.[10]

The list goes on because society is aging. We are living longer but not necessarily healthier.

The consequences of an intensifying chronic disease epidemic are twofold. Firstly, chronic diseases represent a significant burden to those who live with them, as we observed with Simon. Most of us know someone who suffers from diabetes, cardiovascular disease, cancer, or a mental health disorder. The daily experiences of these patients, families, and caregivers who are living and coping with these conditions and their side effects should not be neglected. Secondly, from a systems perspective, managing those diseases puts an ever-growing pressure on total health care expenditures, which in turn makes health care less accessible. In the United States, 90% of the $3.5 trillion annual health care spending is dedicated to chronic and mental health diseases, and this expenditure is projected to continue to outpace gross domestic product growth over the next 15 years.[11] And this upward cost spiral is not unique to the United States.

This unprecedented rise in chronic and mental health diseases, coupled with the continually growing costs that accompany them, require a fundamentally new approach to how we conceptualize and deliver care. What role could DTx play in transforming our health care systems to match the size of this challenge?

Existing Solutions in Health Care Are Not Adopted or Scalable (Enough)

New health care delivery models are emerging. Compared to established pathways, they are more data-driven and rely to a greater degree on digital biomarkers, digital diagnostics, and DTx to measure, diagnose, monitor, and manage patients' health. As such, some of them are providing an entry for DTx in care circuits in recognition of the potential to fulfill unmet needs and enhance patient-centered care.

Early adopters of new medical technologies believe in the potential of DTx to disrupt traditional and often inefficient health care business models through delivering better clinical outcomes at lower cost while providing a superior patient experience. In fact, DTx are said to be one of the most promising avenues for improving health care provision on a global scale, so much so that some even see them as poised to revolutionize medicine. In our view, they will play an important role in the transformation of our health care systems from "sick care" to "health care" and "people care" that's outcome-driven, evidence-based, and experience-focused.

DTx are certainly not going to be cure-alls for the ailments afflicting global health care systems. Although on one hand they offer great promise, Simon's story of using a DTx to manage his pain symptoms, on the other hand, remains anecdotal. DTx are relatively new to the health care arsenal and still in the early days of commercialization. What this means is that patients and caregivers are more likely to have never heard of such solutions or how they can be helpful. And physicians already struggle with myriad mobile applications, each promising to deliver better health outcomes to their patients, so they may be skeptical to try "yet another app." And who is going to pay for all of these tools anyway?

These considerations give rise to important questions:

- How will DTx be implemented?
- How can DTx adoption be expanded?
- Can we harness DTx to broadly decentralize health care?

Technology Alone Cannot Transform Health Care

Taking a technological innovation all the way to the finish line—the clinic or home—involves a wide range of disciplines and expertise, from behavioral science, design thinking, and software engineering to user experience research, gamification, and health care economics. It also depends on inventors and developers being part of a well-oiled ecosystem whose discrete parts are willing to collaborate, often across value chain segments and even country borders. Thus, realized innovation lies not only in the technology itself, but also in how that technology is tested and commercialized, how patients and physicians are engaged, and how all other stakeholders are partnered. This

Missed Opportunities Will Be Costly

Unlike many customer-facing industries (e.g., hospitality, retail, and banking), which have all been transformed by the adoption of new technologies, health care has been slow to open itself to innovation. One only needs to look at the current state of digitization in the health care industry; patchy solutions notwithstanding, it remains an aspiration. To cite one statistic that speaks to this reality, over 12% of Germany's total health care costs (34 billion euros, or US$40 billion), could have been saved in 2018 if the German health care system had been fully digitized.[12] Where would the largest savings and impact have come from? The switch to paperless data via electronic health records (EHRs), which were in fact developed in the 1980s.

EHR systems, like many health technologies (including DTx), belong to the category of innovations presenting important potential benefits. However, their mainstreaming in routine clinical settings remains difficult. Despite billions in incentives spent on expanding their adoption and use globally, the central question about EHR interoperability across all settings of care has yet to be resolved. Further, we still know too little about how EHRs are being used to improve outcomes while drawing on fewer resources. In fact, one study found that it is the opposite: for every hour of clinical work, physicians spent two hours on clerical or EHR-related tasks.[13]

The EHR example underscores that technology alone, even if successfully operationalized and implemented, does not guarantee wide market adoption. For this reason, DTx entrepreneurs should make sure their innovations effectively bridge the gap between development and commercialization. This book contains actionable strategies on how to achieve this outcome.

---

interactional element is what opens doors and pushes new boundaries in terms of technology implementation that improves lives for patients, caregivers, and communities across the globe while also empowering health care professionals.

The Institute for Digital Medicine (WisDM) of the Yong Loo Lin School of Medicine at the National University of Singapore was established with the mission to harness leading-edge technology and forge mutually supportive partnerships between stakeholders involved in its development and commercialization, in order to drive practice-changing medicine that achieves scalable patient impact. In this journey we are guided by a simple but ambitious goal: to develop a framework for implementing and scaling novel pharmacological and digital interventional technologies into yet-to-come models of care.

Granted, the transformation of our health care system has already been set in motion by advances such as artificial intelligence (AI), telehealth, DNA sequencing, personalized medicine, and DTx. We are already transitioning toward a health care system that is more proactive than reactive, more digital than analog, and more data-driven and personalized than one-size-fits-all; a system that will also be more patient- or user-centric, focused on restoring health to individuals rather than on treating body systems and organs in isolation.

We must recognize, however, that technology alone cannot transform health care. Numerous real-world examples have demonstrated that substantial gaps exist between major capital raises and clinical uptake and reimbursement.[14] Transforming health care is indeed about more than introducing new technology; it is also about improving patient outcomes and doing so at a lower cost than under the status quo.

Patients are not demanding new technologies just for the sake of it. They really just want to feel and get better. They need help to treat and manage their conditions, but the *how*—whether by taking a pill, using a mobile app, or benefiting from an algorithm—is less important to them than the *what*, which is the final outcome. Technology should seamlessly integrate into their day-to-day lives, to deliver both a seamless experience and improved quality of life.

Physicians also don't need technology just for the sake of it; what they need is better support to manage their patients in a more individualized way. This can potentially be achieved via access to more granular information that lets them continuously optimize patient care. "It is not because you have an algorithm that you have a commercial-ready product," says Dr. Carolyn Lam, cofounder of the Singaporean medtech company Us2.ai, which uses machine learning to automate the analysis of echocardiograms. "We should not underestimate the amount of work that it takes to integrate with existing EHRs, fix data silos, design the right interface, protect patient data, get all the regulatory approvals, et cetera. It is equally demanding, if not more demanding than it is to develop a new technology," she tells us.

In a nutshell, technology is an enabler but not a solution in and of itself. Getting the technology right is just the beginning of a long and sinuous journey for DTx, often marked by continuous struggles if not outright failure. In reality, a global community of innovators striving to improve patient outcomes are facing the same obstacles. Ultimately, the right innovation blueprint will realize the full potential of DTx.

Who Is This Book For?

In this book, we speak to innovation and business leaders from all corners of the health care universe who are involved in designing and building tomorrow's DTx. They include clinicians, researchers, engineers, patients, startup founders and corporate executives—all driven to ultimately improve patient health outcomes.

DTx represent a convergence point of three different worlds: health care, technology, and business. Developing and commercializing a DTx solution requires a deep understanding of each of these different universes and their vernacular. Which language do you speak?

- *If you "speak" health care*, you may be a clinician, nurse, service lead, or hospital administrator. As such, you understand patients' needs and frustrations, as well as the infrastructural challenges of providing quality patient care under the status quo. You could envision a new DTx solution to benefit your patients (and potentially your practice). The next steps you will need to address is how you develop a DTx technology that embodies your idea while also ensuring viability in practice.
- *If you "speak" technology*, you may be a software developer, engineer, data specialist, or chief technology officer. As such,

you approach the development of DTx in the context of technical performance, including things like processing speed, software architecture, how much computing power it consumes, and maybe even cybersecurity. You may also be thinking about how to properly determine its effectiveness. In order to be useful, however, a health care technology must be successfully taken out of development, established with evidence, and ultimately implemented.

- *If you "speak" business*, you may be an entrepreneur, corporate executive, C-suite leader, or an investor. You likely work in a field such as marketing, advertising, finance, sales, or management. When you think about DTx, you understand the need to size up an opportunity, to evaluate its potential impact on the end users, and to anticipate challenges involved in implementing a new solution in the current health care ecosystem. Successfully addressing financial return and scalability in the DTx journey ahead will be essential.

Realizing Medicine 4.0

This book serves as a blueprint to bring digital therapy to fruition and as a gateway to inspiring unprecedented broader impact on the future of medicine. We therefore aim to offer an end-to-end roadmap for DTx solution scalability that will ultimately help DTx innovators and entrepreneurs deliver impact at scale. Our perspectives and insights come from both academia and the technology industry, including stories and learnings that address the practical realities of DTx development and implementation. We also look within the health care industry for guidance on successful implementation in the clinical setting. Lastly, we take a look at existing as well as aspiring DTx innovations and learn from both their successes and failures.

Along with the frameworks, tools, and insights this book contains, it will prepare you for the inevitable twists and pivots your organization may experience as it gears up for entering the DTx space. It may not provide all the answers, but we hope it will give you a solid foundation for derisking your journey ahead.

After introducing what DTx are and what's unique about them (part I), we explore the main challenges and opportunities for each key development phase of DTx organizations, from the inception of the organization and exploration of potential concepts (part II), to validation of the DTx solution in routine clinical care (part III), and finally the go-to-market strategy and how to deliver impact at scale (part IV).

Part I: What Are Digital Therapeutics? As a new technology, it may be unclear what DTx are and what makes them unique. DTx should not be confused with wellness apps. The distinction between the two is clearly defined by the level of clinical evidence, real-world outcomes, and regulatory oversight involved in their development and evaluation. After reading this first chapter, innovators and business leaders curious about the future of medicine will understand the critically important role of DTx toward changing the way that medicine is practiced.

Part II: The Right Tool for the Right Problem. DTx are a versatile class of medical tools that offer a range of benefits. What kinds of problems are they best positioned to address? In chapters 2–5, we invite readers to develop their thinking about DTx across three dimensions: clinical needs, stakeholders, and venture viability.

Part III: From Pilot to Production. Exploring the real-world potential of DTx is about testing how well they operate in routine clinical practice. During this stage, DTx transition from invention to innovation if their creators are able to demonstrate they represent a solution in day-to-day clinical care. This phase is a litmus test before scale-up and chapters 6–10 guide DTx innovators through the complexities of implementation and adoption of DTx to arrive at the right solution-market fit.

Part IV: Paths to Commercialization. Having a good, tested idea and a minimally viable product do not guarantee commercial success. How do you reach the end users (patients)? How much should you charge for your digital solution? In the final two chapters we explore the importance of having the right strategic partner to distribute and commercialize your DTx and discuss monetization strategies.

Introducing the Key Contributors

This book goes beyond our team's experience in developing and implementing new technologies in health care. It is the result of a collaborative approach that also leverages the experience and know-how of many external distinguished experts in fields such as AI and implementation science. We are privileged to share their thoughts with our readers.

Listed in order of appearance in the book:

Dr. Jessica SHULL
Head of Digital Therapeutics at Vicore Pharma, Sweden
What Are Digital Therapeutics?, page 19

Dr. Jessica Shull is Head of Digital Therapeutics at Vicore Pharma in Sweden. Previously, she led the European Policy work for the Digital Therapeutics Alliance and managed clinical projects for respiratory disease at Bellvitge Hospital in Barcelona.

With 20 years' experience in digital health—from developing virtual surgery devices to integrating digital frameworks at the World Health Organization and at national level—she is now focused on developing digital therapeutics products.

Dr. Ester YEOH
Senior consultant endocrinologist at Admiralty Medical Centre and Khoo Teck Puat Hospital, Singapore
Addressing Unmet Stakeholder Needs, page 43

Dr. Ester Yeoh is trained in endocrinology and internal medicine, with subspecialty interest in type 1 diabetes and hypoglycemia. She leads the Flexible Insulin Therapy team at the Admiralty Medical Centre's Diabetes Clinic, which cares for people with type 1 diabetes.

The team comprises a dietician, diabetes nurse educators, and a health psychologist.

Dr. Yeoh firmly believes in patient education and in empowering her patients with the knowledge and tools to improve diabetes self-management. She has special interests in patient education, mental health in diabetes, and diabetes technologies such as insulin pumps, glucose sensors, and other digital health solutions.

Dr. Raj KUMAR
CEO of UCSI Blue Ocean Strategy Consulting, Malaysia
Addressing Unmet Stakeholder Needs, page 43

Dr. Raj Kumar is currently the CEO of UCSI Blue Ocean Strategy Consulting, a consulting firm that specializes in strategic value innovation. He is a certified Blue Ocean Strategy expert whose consulting insights draw on his vast experience, ranging from setting up business operations to strategic planning, innovation, and project execution.

Dr. Kumar has helped implement Blue Ocean Strategy for international firms, billion-dollar conglomerates, and government agencies. He has also conducted programs on Blue Ocean Strategy across North America, the Middle East, Africa, and the Asia Pacific region, interacting with participants from over 25 countries.

Fabien SOUILLARD
Type 1 diabetes patient, France
Addressing Unmet Stakeholder Needs, page 43

Fabien Souillard was diagnosed with type 1 diabetes when he was 13 years old. Ten years later, after countless consultations with endocrinologists and other physicians, he still struggles with daily finger pricks, carbohydrate counting, and trying his best to have the semblance of a "normal" life. He often needs to visit hospitals and manage his hemoglobin A1c, stomach cramps, and other complications that arise from his condition.

Dr. Robyn MILDON
Founding Executive Director of the Centre for Evidence and
Implementation, Australia
Recommendations for DTx Implementation, page 162

Dr. Robyn Mildon is an internationally recognized authority in the
fields of implementation science, evidence synthesis, and knowledge
translation, as well as program and policy evaluations in health, education, and human services. She is an adjunct associate professor at
Monash University, a visiting professor at the Yong Loo Lin School of
Medicine, codirector of the recently established the Centre for Behavioural and Implementation Science Interventions at the National
University of Singapore, and the inaugural cochair of the Knowledge
Translation and Implementation Group with the Campbell Collaboration, an international systematic review group.

Over her career, Dr. Mildon has helped to advance the implementation of better evidence in policy and practice settings and to improve the quality and effectiveness of health, education, and human
services.

Dr. Kee Yuan NGIAM
Group Chief Technology Officer, National University Health System,
Singapore; Deputy Chief Medical Informatics Officer, National
University Hospital, Singapore
Recommendations for DTx Implementation, "What Health Care System
Managers Expect," page 162

Dr. Kee Yuan Ngiam is the Group Chief Technology Officer of the
National University Health System (NUHS) Singapore, overseeing
the technology deployment in the Western health care cluster. In this
role he assists the system's chief executive to implement new technologies throughout the NUHS and serves as chief advisor to the NUHS
Centre for Innovation in Healthcare. Dr. Ngiam is concurrently the
Deputy Chief Medical Informatics Officer of NUHS, with a special
focus on artificial intelligence research and implementation in health
care. In his capacity as assistant professor of surgery at the Yong Loo

Lin School of Medicine at the National University of Singapore, he also engages in research into endocrine and metabolic surgery.

Dr. Ngiam led the operationalization of the DISCOVERY AI platform—a translational research-to-production AI platform that is the basis for operational validation of advanced deep-learning AI models—by encouraging collaboration between computer scientists and clinicians. Since its launch, the platform has promoted interdisciplinary collaborations, reducing the time to translation and accelerating the pace of health care innovation.

Christopher HARDESTY

Partner, Pureland Venture, Singapore
Paths to Commercialization, page 191

Christopher Hardesty specializes in building early-stage medical innovations for scale-up in Asia and beyond. He has lived and worked in more than 50 countries to design public-private health system financial schemes, including for the creation of pathways for adoption of medical innovations. He is also a member of KPMG's Global Healthcare & Life Sciences Centre of Excellence and engages in adjunct lecturing, research/writing, and startup/fund advisory so as to be a steward of innovation acceleration across the health care ecosystem.

Dr. Eddie MARTUCCI

Cofounder and CEO of Akili Interactive Labs, United States
Conclusion. The Future of DTx, page 249

Dr. Eddie Martucci is a cofounder and CEO of Akili Interactive Labs. After earning his doctorate, he studied health care entrepreneurship as a Kauffman Fellow through support from the Kauffman Foundation, a nationally recognized leadership program for venture capitalists and innovators. For the last 11 years, Dr. Martucci has worked at Boston-based PureTech Health, a health care biotech company, where he helped launch their digital health initiative and cofounded two health-focused startups. In 2012, he cofounded and currently serves as CEO for Akili Interactive Labs, a company recognized as pioneering the new field of "digital medicine."

Matt OON

Founder and CEO of Acceset, Singapore

Appendix B. How to Translate Evidence-Based Theories to the Design of Digitally Delivered Mental Health Interventions, page 270

Matt Oon is the founder of Acceset (pronounced "asset"), a social enterprise platform that aims to transform and normalize mental health care in Singapore through providing anonymous text-based emotional support for students via a digital letter-writing portal.

Soon after founding the company, Oon received the 2018 Queen's Young Leaders Award in recognition of his commitment to revolutionizing the way we perceive mental health in the twenty-first century. He was a member of the Wellcome Trust Mental Health Science Community, and he was the recipient of the Philip Yeo Initiative fellowship and a member of the Generation T list, both initiatives recognizing leaders of tomorrow who are shaping Asia's future. His work ranges from capacity building, such as the development of empathy skills in students, to translational research work that involves implementing the digital letter-writing platform in schools to better support students.

Finally, this book has also been shaped by input from 70 DTx and digital health CEOs, entrepreneurs, innovators, clinicians, payers, and industry experts across 15 countries in America, Asia, and Europe. We acknowledge the contributions of:

Adrian Ang, AEvice, Singapore
Alexandre Tavares, Novartis, Singapore
Alexandria Marie Remus, N.1 Institute for Health, Singapore
Aline Noizet, Digital Health Connector, Spain
Amir Bozorgzadeh, Virtuleap, Portugal
Anthony Pannozzo, Frog Design, United States
Antonio Estrella, Taliossa, Singapore
Azran Osman-Rani, Naluri, Malaysia
Benjamin Belot, Kurma Partners, France

Carolyn Lam, Us2.ai, Singapore
Charlotte Lee, Big Health, United Kingdom
Christopher Hardesty, Pureland Venture, Singapore
Christopher Lew, Rock Health, United States
Cole Sirucek, DocDoc, Singapore
Craig A. Delarge, The Digital Mental Health Project, United States
Danny Kim, Welt, Korea
Dorothea Koh, Bot MD, Singapore
Edward Booty, reach52, Singapore
Elena Mustatea, Bold Health, United Kingdom
Elizabeth Galbut, SoGal Ventures, United States
Eugene Hong, DBS, Singapore
Francois Cadiou, Healint, Singapore
Gabriel Sim, APACMed, Singapore
Geck Hong Yeo, N.1 Institute for Health, Singapore
Georgios Kaissis, Technical University of Munich, Germany
Girish Bommakanti, Access Health, India
Guillaume Bezie, Sibius, France
Hilary Thomas, KPMG, United Kingdom
Hsien-Hsien Lei, AMCHAM, Singapore
Jennifer Shannon, Cognoa, United States
Jeremy Lim, AMiLi, Singapore
Julian Sham, Amazon Web Services, Singapore
Kitty Lee, Temus, Singapore
Maleena Suppiah Cavert, National University Health System, Singapore
Markus Pratschke, Sandoz, Germany
Melissa Hudzik, Wilson Sonsini Goodrich & Rosati, United States
Miguel Rivera, Novartis, Singapore
Nana Bit-Avragim, iHospital InnoLab, Germany
Nang Duangnapa, Mercer, Singapore
Nawal Roy, Holmusk, Singapore
Neil Narale, Mercer, Singapore
Nicholas Brocklebank, Global Legal Solutions Group, Singapore

Owen McCarthy, MedRhythms, United States
Peta Latimer, Mercer, Singapore
Peter Hawkes, Johnson & Johnson, Singapore
Pierre A. Morgon, MRGN Advisors, Switzerland
Pieu RoyChoudhury, Medtronic, Singapore
Pin Kwok, Savonix, Singapore
Pocket Sun, SoGal Ventures, China
Renato De Giorgi, Axenya, Argentina
Reza Shokri, National University of Singapore
Rohit Bhatia, Cerebral, United States
Sajid Rahman, Digital Healthcare Solutions, Bangladesh
Sean G. Kang, Welt, Korea
Siva Nadarajah, JOGO Health, United States
Smrithi Vijayakumar, N.1 Institute for Health, Singapore
Snehal Patel, MyDoc, Singapore
Sue Anne Toh, NOVI Health, Singapore
Sundeep Lal, BioConnexUS, United States
Sven Jungmann, Founderslane, Germany
Theodore Wonpeum Kee, N.1 Institute for Health, Singapore
Timothy Johns, Department for International Trade, China
Valeria Burrone, MEng, Italy
Viroshini Hari Krishnan, AXA, Singapore
V Vien Lee, N.1 Institute for Health, Singapore
Wai Chiong Loke, Ministry of Health Office for Healthcare
    Transformation, Singapore
Wee Tee Soh, National University Health System, Singapore
William Bao Bean, SOSV, China
Xavier Tadeo, N.1 Institute for Health, Singapore
Zia Zaman, Microsoft, Singapore

NOTES
1. Rubin, "Epidemiology and Risk Factors for Spine Pain."
2. Kaplan at al., *Priority Medicines for Europe and the World: 2013 Update.*
3. Wu et al., "Global Low Back Pain Prevalence and Years Lived with Disability from 1990 to 2017."

4. Hartvigsen et al., "What Low Back Pain Is and Why We Need to Pay Attention."

5. Hajat and Stein, "The Global Burden of Multiple Chronic Conditions"; Buttorff, Ruder, and Bauman, *Multiple Chronic Conditions in the United States.*

6. World Health Organization, "Cardiovascular Diseases (CVDs)."

7. Sherwin et al., "The Prevention or Delay of Type 2 Diabetes."

8. World Health Organization, "Diabetes: Key Facts."

9. Ahmad, Ormiston-Smith, and Sasieni, "Trends in the Lifetime Risk of Developing Cancer in Great Britain."

10. World Health Organization, "Dementia: Key Facts."

11. Centers for Diseases Control and Prevention, "Health and Economic Costs of Chronic Diseases"; Lorenzoni et al., *Health Spending Projections to 2030.*

12. Hehner, Biesdorf, and Möller, "Digitizing Healthcare—Opportunities for Germany."

13. Sinsky et al., "Allocation of Physician Time in Ambulatory Practice."

14. Haimovitch and Kirkner, "A Look Behind Revision Optics' Shuttered Door"; Keown, "Sienna Biopharmaceuticals Files for Bankruptcy, Delaying Phase III Psoriasis Trial"; Reuter, "Proteus Files for Bankruptcy: Where Did It Falter?"

- PART I

WHAT ARE DIGITAL THERAPEUTICS?

CHAPTER 1

Digital Health Solutions versus Digital Therapeutics

This chapter was written with contributions by Dr. Jessica Shull, Head of Digital Therapeutics at Vicore Pharma in Sweden. Previously, she led the European Policy work for Digital Therapeutics Alliance, the global digital therapeutics (DTx) industry association.

Digital health and *digital therapeutics* are popular terms that are often used interchangeably, yet critical distinctions between the two exist. "Digital health," as an umbrella term, encompasses all technologies, platforms, and systems across the wellness and health care industries that engage consumers for lifestyle, wellness, and health-related purposes.[1] It includes all trackers and "quantified self" apps, platforms, or solutions, from such consumer wearables as sleep trackers and fitness apps (e.g., Apple watch, Fitbit's range of fitness products, and the Oura Ring for sleep and activity tracking) to clinically evaluated cardiac health monitors and cloud infrastructures (e.g., BioTelemetry, Coala Heart Monitor, and Philips VitalHealth). Under this concept of digital health, we identify three categories of digital health solutions: wellness and support, diagnostic and monitoring, and digital therapeutics (table 1.1).

Table 1.1. Three categories of digital health solutions

	Wellness and support	Diagnostic and monitoring	Digital therapeutics
Overview	Products that capture, store, and transmit health data	Products that measure and/or intervene	Products that deliver therapeutic interventions directly to patients
Clinical evidence	*Not typically required*	Required	Required
Real-world outcomes	*Not typically required*	*Not typically required*	Required
Regulatory oversight	*Varies depending on the intended use and function of the solution*	Required	Required
Examples	Lifestyle apps and fitness trackers, telehealth platforms, health information technology, consumer health information, enterprise support	Digital diagnostics, digital biomarkers, remote patient monitoring, medication adherence tools, ingestible sensors,[1] connected drug delivery devices	Digital cognitive therapy, digital behavioral therapy, digital physical therapy

Source: Adapted from Digital Therapeutics Alliance, *Ensuring Appropriate Quality, Access, and Utilization of Digital Therapeutics.*

[1] What about wearables and sensors? Additional functionalities, digitally delivered or not, may be required to optimize further patient care and health outcomes, such as wearables and sensors, ingestible or not. These functionalities could be important to the physicians to assess and optimize overall therapy (e.g., clinical decision support system or face-to-face education and training). On their own, these components can't be considered DTx, but they could be important elements to the DTx's overall value proposition and market success.

As an independent category within digital health, the appeal of digital therapeutics, or DTx, lies in blending patient-centric technologies with evidence-based medicine to treat, manage, and prevent a broad spectrum of chronic conditions and disorders. According to Click Therapeutics, which develops and commercializes digital medical treatments, the term "digital therapeutics" was coined in 2012, the same year their company was founded (so they would know). Back then, it was defined as "outcomes-based mobile software," quite similar to its current definition by Pear Therapeutics—another DTx player that develops prescription-based digital interventions—as "software-based disease treatments."

The nonprofit trade association Digital Therapeutics Alliance (DTA) characterizes DTx as follows:[2]

DTx deliver therapeutic interventions[3] directly to patients . . . [that] may be used independently or in tandem with remote or in-person clinician-delivered therapy to optimize patient outcomes. . . . Digital therapeutics undergo clinical trials, collect real-world outcomes, and are based on patient-centered core principles and product development best practices, including product design, usability, data security, and privacy standards. . . .

> *What value could DTx products bring to this situation?*

- Increase remote access to therapies that are clinically demonstrated as safe and effective.
- Provide care independent of a patient's schedule and in the safety of their home environment.
- Are easily scalable and often accessible through patient-owned devices (e.g., smartphones, tablets).
- Generate actionable, real-world insights that enable intelligent data-driven care management and clinical decision making.

Similarly, DTx must also adhere to ten foundational principles:[4]

- Prevent, manage, or treat a medical disorder or disease
- Produce a medical intervention that is driven by software
- Incorporate design, manufacture, and quality best practices
- Engage end users in product development and usability processes
- Incorporate patient privacy and security protections
- Apply product deployment, management, and maintenance best practices
- Publish trial results inclusive of clinically meaningful outcomes in peer-reviewed journals
- Be reviewed and cleared or approved by regulatory bodies as required to support product claims of risk, efficacy, and intended use
- Make claims appropriate to clinical evaluation and regulatory status
- Collect, analyze, and apply real-world evidence and/or product performance data

In a nutshell, DTx are a subset of digital health that is based on clinical evidence, generate real-world outcomes, and are subject to regulatory oversight.

How Do DTx Work in Practice?

To understand how DTx work in practice, let's look at diabetes, one of the top 10 causes of death globally,[5] as an example. You probably don't need to be convinced about the burden diabetes represents to patients, families, and our health care systems. Patients with type 1 or type 2 diabetes often struggle with managing their condition, and this is especially true in the months after they are diagnosed, when the vast majority of them experience difficulties with keeping their blood glucose level below recommended thresholds.[6] This is a problem waiting for a DTx solution.

Granted, there are myriad of mobile applications with various features for diabetes management that are now available, each offering a mix of such functionalities as food diaries, calorie counters, and weight management programs. A few of these apps, however, have been developed using evidence-based frameworks (appendix B) and would therefore not be considered digital therapeutics. BlueStar®,[7] a software program powered by Welldoc and cleared by the US Food and Drug Administration (FDA) as a Class II medical device for diabetes, is one of the exceptions.

DTx Case Study: BlueStar®

BlueStar®, an AI-driven DTx solution available as a mobile app (figure 1.1) and a web version, offers users advanced coaching and tailored guidance for managing diabetes, including medication administration, physical activity, smart food choices, and psychosocial well-being.

Since its launch in 2013, the platform offers a robust set of capabilities for type 1 and type 2 diabetes management. For example, a patient can use the insulin dose calculator to find out the exact dose of bolus

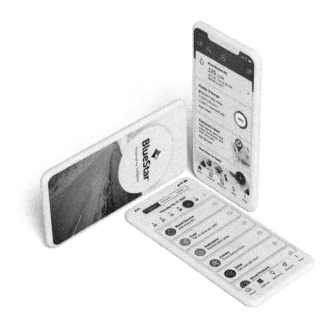

FIGURE 1.1. Overview of BlueStar's mobile app. Source: Photo by Welldoc Inc., 2022

insulin they should take for a given carbohydrates intake amount or blood glucose value. The platform can also analyze and report blood glucose test results and support medication adherence by providing coaching messages (motivational, behavioral, and educational) based on real-time blood glucose values and trends.

As a result, based on individual readings, patients are gently "nudged" by a selection of more than 30,000 automated, tailored coaching messages to take the most appropriate medication, diet, or exercise-related action, driven by clinical and evidence-based guidelines.[8] The compatibility of BlueStar® with a number of blood glucose monitoring and continuous glucose monitoring devices, blood pressure cuffs, and weight scales further facilitates its seamless integration into a patient's day-to-day lifestyle.

Since using the BlueStar® app does not require a prescription, the company is working closely with payers and employers so current and future users can have access to the app directly through their health plans and wellness programs—although a journey with BlueStar® can also start with a physician recommending it.

In 2020, the FDA cleared BlueStar's Insulin Adjustment Program (IAP), a novel medical prescription (Rx) feature that supports individuals with type 2 diabetes using long-acting insulin. Patients who are specifically prescribed IAP, in addition to the basic BlueStar® platform, are guided through the process of basal insulin titration and benefit from the ease of real-time adjustments to their insulin without having to use a calculator. Insulin initiation and titration require a lot of effort and adjustments from patients and their health care providers, so this advanced insulin calibration feature fills an important need. Concretely, health care providers use a web interface to prescribe an initial dose and "BlueStar® does the rest."[9] It also allows physicians, diabetes educators, and care coordinators to follow the evolution and progress of their patients through their own dashboards and intervene in a highly targeted way when a situation of risk has been flagged by the system. This is an example of a digital therapeutic intervention delivered directly to patients.

Diabetes solutions with BlueStar® Rx is just one example of how DTx can help patients in managing their conditions and health care professionals in remote monitoring their patients. Fortunately, the therapeutic areas, applications, and opportunities for DTx go beyond diabetes and these technologies can be used in a range of clinical indications, including for pain, attention deficit disorder, mental health disorders, and cancer assistive therapy at various stages of development and regulatory clearance (table 1.2).

According to their mechanism of action, DTx can be further subdivided into two broad categories:

- DTx used as *standalone treatments* (a.k.a. drug-replacement therapies) and
- DTx used *in conjunction with other therapies* (a.k.a. adjunctive digital therapies, companion digital therapies, or drug-plus DTx) to augment their effectiveness, such as BlueStar's AI-guided insulin adjustment program.

Table 1.2. Selected examples of well-known DTx solutions

Companies and therapeutic areas	DTx solutions	Selected outcomes
Akili Interactive: Attention deficit hyperactivity disorder (ADHD)	Utilizing adaptive sensory stimulus software for the treatment of ADHD delivered through a captivating and engaging video game experience.	Indicated to improve attention function as measured by computer-based testing.[1]
Big Health: Sleep improvement program	Sleepio is a digital sleep improvement program based on digital cognitive behavioral therapy (dCBT) to help overcome poor sleep and thereby improve mental health.	76% of long-term poor sleepers achieve healthy sleep.[2]
BlueStar®: Diabetes (metabolism)	BlueStar® combines individual patient treatment data with machine learning algorithms to provide tailored motivational, behavioral, and educational coaching messages to aid in diabetes self-management.	A 1.7- to 2.0-point mean A1c reduction for adults living with type 2 diabetes who used BlueStar® as well as a savings, on average, from US$254 to US$271 per user per month.[3]
Click Therapeutics: Smoking cessation	DTx-as-a-service solution builder for biopharma companies, leveraging the company's Click Neurobehavioral Intervention Platform. It has a pipeline of other DTx for a variety of indications. Clickotine, the most advanced one, is a clinically validated fully digital smoking cessation program.	45.2% of the participants (n = 188) had stopped smoking at the end of the study.[4]
Kaia Health: Musculoskeletal disorders	Delivery of physical exercises, behavioral therapy, and education for chronic back pain patients, to help both the body and the brain cope with musculoskeletal conditions. The company also has a DTx for pulmonary rehabilitation.	Users report an average pain level decrease of 43% over 12 weeks.[5]
MedRhythms: Neurologic disease and injury	Neurologic music therapy to address motor, speech, and cognitive dysfunction caused by neurologic disease or injury.	A single, fully automated training visit resulted in increased usual and fast walking speeds.[6]
Pear Therapeutics: Substance use disorder[7]	Prescription DTx to treat patients suffering from a range of serious diseases, including substance use disorder (SUD), opioid use disorder (OUD), and chronic insomnia.	Patients in recovery from SUD, whose primary substance of abuse was not opioids, were more than two times as likely to abstain from drug use when reSET was added to outpatient therapy versus when it was not.[8]

(continued)

Table 1.2. (continued)

Companies and therapeutic areas	DTx solutions	Selected outcomes
Voluntis: Cancer	Oleena's algorithms serve cancer patients by providing personalized guidance on how best to mitigate symptoms, using on-demand directions for initiation and dosing of supportive therapies based on the patient's individual care plan. It also provides patient monitoring and generates insights for the care team.	More effective communication between patients and health care providers; personalized supportive care plan for better adherence and outcomes.

Note: DTx companies listed in alphabetical order.

[1] Akili Interactive, "Akili Announces FDA Clearance of EndeavorRx for Children with ADHD, the First Prescription Treatment Delivered through a Video Game."

[2] Espie et al., "A Randomized, Placebo-Controlled Trial of Online Cognitive Behavioral Therapy for Chronic Insomnia Disorder Delivered via an Automated Media-Rich Web Application."

[3] Welldoc Inc., "WellDoc Validates Potential of Its Digital Therapeutic, BlueStar, to Significantly Reduce Healthcare Costs."

[4] Iacoviello et al., "Clickotine, a Personalized Smartphone App for Smoking Cessation."

[5] Toelle et al., "App-Based Multidisciplinary Back Pain Treatment versus Combined Physiotherapy Plus Online Education."

[6] Hutchinson et al., "A Music-Based Digital Therapeutic: Proof-of-Concept Automation of a Progressive and Individualized Rhythm-Based Walking Training Program after Stroke."

[7] Before this book's publication, Pear Therapeutics began a reorganization.

[8] Pear Therapeutics, "Reset for Recovery: The Proof." Accessed November, 11, 2022. https://www.resetforrecovery.com/reset#the-proof.

So how exactly do digital therapeutics differ from digital health overall? Below we outline three essential advantages that distinguish DTx from the broad mix of digital health inventions.

DTx Differential Advantage #1: Clinical Evidence at the Personal Level

Within the digital therapeutic concept, *therapeutic* is an important word. It refers to the intended use of the digital solution and highlights the fact that there is clinical grade evidence backing up its safety and efficacy, two critical aspects of any therapy that are demonstrated traditionally in randomized clinical trials (RCTs). Health care providers weighing the option of recommending or prescribing a DTx to their patients should always read carefully the product label, whose importance is "paramount, because it's the sacred communication that the company can make to the prescribing clinicians, and it defines if the product is safe, efficacious and may provide benefits to the patients," suggests Corey M. McCann, president and CEO of Pear Therapeutics.[10]

Indeed, the level of clinical evidence is of utmost importance here as it is what differentiates DTx from other digital health solutions. The latter kind may indirectly lead to clinical benefits, but they are not subjected to clinical trials as per regulation by specific countries. On the contrary, Pear Therapeutics's reSET and reSET-O first products, cleared by the FDA, have been tested and validated in six RCTs involving over 1,500 patients diagnosed with substance use disorder.[11]

According to the levels of evidence used to rank the quality of medical and health care research, RCTs and systematic reviews of RCTs remain the gold standard for evaluating the effectiveness of interventions, including DTx. This hierarchy provides guidance about the types of evidence that are more likely to provide trustworthy answers to the clinical questions we are trying to answer. For instance, if we look at the potential treatment benefits of DTx in answering the question "Does this intervention help?," findings from an RCT will be of level 2 (with level 1 being the highest and level 5 being the lowest), while those from a systematic review of RCTs or of N-of-1 trials will be of level 1.[12]

Although both RCTs and N-of-1 trials are necessary, some research requires trial designs that are difficult to implement in practice or that make difficult data standardization afterward. Suffice it to say that these challenges are surmountable and even play a role in driving clinical trial design innovation.

DTx Differential Advantage #2: Real-World Evidence Generation

Evidence of the benefits of DTx may come not only from clinical trials, but also from what we call real-world evidence (RWE). By design, DTx have the capacity to collect and analyze, in real or near-real time, extremely valuable real-world data (RWD) about a patient's current state of health. Such data provide researchers and health technology assessment specialists with powerful insights relating to the usage, benefits, and risks of an intervention that conventional drugs, devices, and treatments usually can't give. As any clinician will tell you, RWD are crucial for treatment decisions, since they provide an additional understanding of treatment risks and benefits in routine clinical practice, in contrast to evidence generated under the highly controlled conditions of clinical trials.

To put this into perspective, we know that often clinical trial participants are not representative of real-world patients.[13] Sometimes this may be due to cohort size (about 60% of trials enroll 100 or fewer subjects[14]), a lack of gender and racial diversity, overly restrictive eligibility criteria (i.e., frequent exclusion of elderly patients and patients with comorbidities), or selection bias that favors positive results (i.e., recruitment of predominantly young healthy people). The implication of such enrollment practices is that trials may exclude many patients seen in everyday clinical practice, thereby limiting the applicability of RCT findings to usual care settings and reinforcing the importance of RWE.

> Real-world evidence is of greatest importance since clinical trials are only as good as they have been designed and may not reflect the true effectiveness of a solution in the real world. You have for example overly restrictive eligibility criteria, such as those of a recent trial assessing a DTx, which excluded patients who couldn't commit to spending 40 minutes a day on their smartphone for 7 days a week. That's not what DTx are designed for or how they are intended to be used or fit in patients' day-to-day life.[15]   —Ken Cahill, CEO and cofounder of SilverCloud Health

Due to the dynamic nature of the DTx development process in response to new data, DTx are also particularly well-suited for leveraging RWD to continuously improve how interventions are designed and delivered. The aim of such iterative fine-tuning—sometimes achieved by human engineers and sometimes by reinforcement machine-learning algorithms—is to optimize clinical outcomes. In this sense, the capacity of DTx to generate RWE complementary to evidence generated in clinical trials and to feed it back to improve the technology is particularly important. This is because all stakeholders, from patients to physicians to regulators,[16] are intrinsically interested in understanding how DTx can deliver value above and beyond conventional therapies and other digital health applications.

DTx Differential Advantage #3: Regulatory Oversight

There is a clear line separating how pharmaceutical drugs and supplements are marketed and used. As a consumer, you surely would have seen on supplements' labels the message "This statement has not been evaluated by the FDA. This product is not intended to diagnose, treat, cure, or prevent any disease." The reasons are simple: supplements, unlike drugs, don't have to demonstrate their safety or effectiveness before reaching the market, don't require post-marketing surveillance, don't follow pharmaceutical good manufacturing practices, and their manufacturers are not allowed to make disease treatment claims. In essence, as supplements are not intended for medical use, they are not regulated in the same manner.[17]

Just as pharmaceutical drugs are distinct from supplements because of stringent regulatory requirements they must meet before being marketed, DTx are distinct from digital health solutions in general. Namely, DTx are commonly regulated under the software as a medical device (SaMD) framework developed by the International Medical Device Regulators Forum. This means that DTx must comply with regulatory requirements for software medical devices throughout their entire life cycle, starting from product development all the way to post-market monitoring and surveillance following product introduction.[18]

Even still, the traditional paradigm of medical device regulation was developed specifically with medical devices in mind and as such does not fully cover the unique characteristics of DTx. This necessarily presents limitations when using SaMD to evaluate such novel technologies. To respond to this new set of challenges and to the growing interest in using DTx in clinical practice, national authorities and payers have started introducing innovative regulatory approaches that will likely eventually converge around new standards across countries. As of 2022 we have observed several different approaches:

- In **Singapore**: Currently DTx fall under the definition of medical devices and as such are regulated by the Health Sciences Authority (HSA) under the Health Products Act.[19] Conscious of the complexities and challenges of incorporating emerging new technologies, such as artificial intelligence applications intended to be used for medical purposes, the HSA recently issued guidelines to provide clarity on the regulatory requirements for software medical devices throughout their entire life cycle from product development all the way to post-market surveillance.[20]

  Recently, Biofourmis, which is focused on predictive care, obtained HSA approval for its two AI-based platforms: Biovitals

Analytics Engine, which enables constant monitoring of individual patients' physiology-based health data, and Rhythm-Analytics, which provides automated interpretation of cardiac arrhythmias. The digital therapeutic reSET from Pear Therapeutics was also the first HSA-authorized prescription DTx to be available in Singapore in 2020.

- In **Germany**: At the end of 2019, Germany launched its Digital Healthcare Act, introducing the concept of "app on prescription" as part of health care provided to patients. Under this new legislation, physicians and psychotherapists can prescribe digital health applications (*digitale Gesundheitsanwendungen*, or DiGA for short).[21] To get on the list of approved and reimbursable apps, these solutions need to successfully pass the assessment of Germany's Federal Institute for Drugs and Medical Devices. The entire process from filing to approval has been designed to be a fast-track process that can be completed within just three months. As of March 2023, over 500 DiGA applications had been submitted to the institute for review, 28 DiGAs had been provisionally approved, and 16 had been permanently approved.[22] Following Germany's lead, other reimbursement pathways are emerging in Europe (e.g., France, Belgium, UK, Italy).
- In the **European Union**: The eHealth Stakeholder Group, the European Commission's expert group on European digital health policy, published *Proposed Guiding Principles for Reimbursement of Digital Health Products and Solutions*. This document intends to help member states' authorities "to modernise national reimbursement and financing schemes for the purpose of enabling digital transformation in EU healthcare systems."[23]
- In the **United Kingdom**: In early 2020, the National Health Service (NHS) published a draft version of its *Digital Health Technology Standard* (DHTS),[24] which aims to accelerate how digital health technologies are reviewed, commissioned, and scaled for use across the wider health and care system, as well

as to provide guidance to digital health technology developers. The DHTS focuses particularly on requirements and safeguards that cover data-driven technology solutions, the development and design of such solutions, and the regulatory framework that ensures data protection and security. Public insurance coverage is decided by local NHS organizations, such as the 43 existing Integrated Care Systems. Additionally, the NHS has negotiated licensing agreements with selected DTx developers, allowing for free-of-charge DTx available in the NHS app library.

- In the **United States**: In 2017, the FDA launched the Digital Health Software Precertification (Pre-Cert) Program as the agency's response to an increasingly complex digital health ecosystem powered by fast-paced technological innovation. The program aims to provide more streamlined and efficient regulatory oversight of software-based medical devices developed by DTx manufacturers who have demonstrated a robust culture of quality and organizational excellence, as well as commitment to monitoring the real-world performance of their products once they are commercialized in the US market. DTx inclusion in corporative benefit packages and private health insurance schemes is growing, and some Medicare and Medicaid programs guarantee public insurance coverage of DTx.[25]

These regulatory advances reflect the multifaceted transformation of traditional models of medical care, self-management, and prevention propelled by DTx. For the time being, however, DTx organizations need to navigate an uncertain and evolving regulatory space and manage unclear business risks, such as the time required to bring a DTx to the market, and challenges, such as those linked to reimbursement.

Earlier in this chapter while introducing digital therapeutics, we emphasized the importance of the word *therapeutic*. Before we conclude, we would also like to highlight the importance of the word *digital*. DTx deliver evidence-based therapeutic interventions that aim to positively influence patients' health status or behavior, with the primary

Key Takeaways

In addition to drugs and medical devices, physicians can now prescribe digital therapeutic (DTx) solutions, either as a standalone treatment or in tandem with current therapy options, to achieve improved health outcomes. As a category, DTx are a subset of digital health, grounded in clinical evidence and compliant with regulatory requirements. Due to their capability to deliver software-based disease treatments (via a program, application, or platform), they should not be confused with digital wellness and lifestyle apps, which cannot and do not make treatment claims. A useful analogy that illustrates the difference between DTx and digital health is the distinction between pharmaceutical drugs (FDA-cleared and -regulated) and supplements (unregulated).

mechanism of action being performed *digitally*. In essence, DTx innovations are made possible thanks to advances in technology with the potential to change the way researchers assess clinical effectiveness (chapter 7), the way regulators exercise regulatory oversight and, put simply, the way health professionals provide health care.

In conclusion, DTx are by nature patient-focused solutions, designed to be used directly by patients or their caregivers, such as parents of children diagnosed with ADHD using Akili Interactive's solution EndeavorRx. They offer the possibility to change the course of disease throughout the care continuum, from diagnosis[26] and early detection to management and treatment of medical disorders, including the possibility to optimize the effects of medication. Ultimately, DTx aim to improve patient health outcomes by enabling more individualized and continuous care, while leaning on the best available evidence. In this book we will walk you through examples and evolutions that show how the combination at scale of technology with evidence-based medicine has the revolutionary potential to transform personalized patient care.[27]

NOTES

1. Digital Therapeutics Alliance, *Digital Health Industry Categorization.*

2. Digital Therapeutics Alliance, "Finding Value in Digital Therapeutics during COVID-19."

3. Intervention is the main reason why, in the potential absence of real-world outcomes, diagnostics and monitoring differ from DTx. Solutions for symptoms monitoring (e.g., COVID-19 symptom monitoring), medication adherence tools (e.g., smart pill bottles or dispensers), or ingestible sensors (e.g., the now-defunct Proteus) are not considered DTx as these solutions track and monitor but do not aim to alter patients' states or behaviors. There is no intervention.

4. Digital Therapeutics Alliance, *Digital Therapeutics Definition and Core Principles.*

5. World Health Organization, "The Top 10 Causes of Death."

6. Fiagbe et al., "Prevalence of Controlled and Uncontrolled Diabetes Mellitus."

7. BlueStar® and BlueStar® Rx are registered trademarks of Welldoc Inc.

8. Digital Therapeutics Alliance, "DTx Product Profile: BlueStar."

9. Welldoc Inc., "Welldoc Receives FDA Clearance for Long-Acting Insulin Support for Award-Winning Digital Health Solution BlueStar."

10. Corey M. McCann, "Emerging Prescription Digital Therapeutics" (presentation, APACMed Virtual Forum, Singapore, September 24, 2020).

11. Pear Therapeutics, "Pear Therapeutics Closes $20 Million Financing."

12. OCEBM Levels of Evidence Working Group, "The Oxford 2011 Levels of Evidence."

13. Kennedy-Martin et al., "A Literature Review on the Representativeness of Randomized Controlled Trial Samples and Implications for the External Validity of Trial Results."

14. Califf et al., "Characteristics of Clinical Trials Registered in ClinicalTrials .gov, 2007–2010."

15. Ken Cahill, "Emerging Prescription Digital Therapeutics" (presentation, APACMed Virtual Forum, Singapore, September 24, 2020).

16. US Food and Drug Administration, *Use of Real-World Evidence to Support Regulatory Decision-Making for Medical Devices.*

17. Although supplements do not need FDA safety and performance approvals before commercialization, manufacturers and distributors are "responsible for evaluating the safety and labeling of their products before marketing to ensure that they meet all the requirements of the Federal Food, Drug, and Cosmetic Act as amended by DSHEA and FDA regulations," and the "FDA has the authority to take action against any adulterated or misbranded dietary supplement product after it reaches the market" (US Food and Drug Administration, "Dietary Supplements," accessed April 4, 2022, https://www.fda.gov/food/dietary-supplements).

18. Health Sciences Authority, *Regulatory Guidelines for Software Medical Devices: A Lifecycle Approach.*

19. Singapore Statutes Online, "Health Products Act 2007."

20. Health Sciences Authority, *Regulatory Guidelines for Software Medical Devices*.

21. A Digital Health Application is defined by the Digital Supply Act (DVG) in Germany as a medical device with the following characteristics: Medical device of risk class I or IIa (according to MDR or, within the framework of the transitional regulations, according to MDD); The main function of DiGA is based on digital technologies; the medical purpose is essentially achieved by the main digital function; The DiGA supports the detection, monitoring, treatment or alleviation of diseases or the detection, treatment, alleviation or compensation of injuries or disabilities; The DiGA is used by the patient or by the service provider and the patient together.

22. Roehl, "DiGA: Digital Therapeutics in Germany"; Bundesinstitut für Arzneimittel und Medizinprodukte [Federal Institute for Drugs and Medical Devices], DiGA-Verzeichnis [DiGA directory], accessed April 4, 2022. https://diga.bfarm.de/de/verzeichnis.

23. eHealth Stakeholder Group, *Proposed Guiding Principles for Reimbursement of Digital Health Products and Solutions*, 5.

24. Joyce, *NHS Digital Health Technology Standard*.

25. Ravot and Ascione, "Access/Reimbursement Policies for Digital Therapeutics Already in Use in National Health Systems"; Digital Therapeutics Alliance. "DTx by Country."

26. It's important to note that according to the Digital Healthcare Act in Germany, solutions aimed at primary prevention of disease are not considered DTx. To be considered DTx, an application should contribute to preventing the worsening of an already diagnosed disease (secondary prevention) or of a secondary disease or complication (tertiary prevention).

27. Evidence-based medicine is defined as "the conscientious, explicit and judicious use of current best evidence in making decisions about the care of individual patients" (Szajewska, "Evidence-Based Medicine and Clinical Research," 14).

PART II

THE RIGHT TOOL FOR THE RIGHT PROBLEM

All too often in the technology world we encounter examples of a technology solution looking for a problem. But the best and most useful innovations—in health care or elsewhere—result from identifying and defining the problem first and growing a solution from there. If one is looking at a problem from a single vantage point (e.g., from a technologist's or clinician's perspective), it is easy to overlook important aspects of building a thoughtfully designed and scalable business while keeping the end user in sight at all times. As you, our reader, may be eager to get a promising DTx technology built, a first pilot study running, or a first round of funding secured, there is a risk you may be so focused on operational details that you are missing the forest for the trees. In this first part of the book, we delve into the details of venture formation. We offer you three perspectives to help you make sure you are solving the right problem and equip you with the knowledge to overcome common challenges faced by DTx organizations at the initial stage.

Checklists save lives. That's the powerful message the World Health Organization championed back in 2008 to encourage surgeons across the world to use checklists when they operate as a way to guarantee safety and avoid costly mistakes.[1] Checklists can also save emerging organizations from pitfalls that can cost them their businesses. As you gear up for your DTx development journey (or even if the idea is still just a seed in your mind), we invite you to consider the items on the following checklist. They are intended to serve as a balcony from which you can view and assess the progress of your venture down on the ground, preemptively recognize challenges that lie ahead, and take timely or corrective action as you advance your idea. Building a DTx is an iterative process, so be sure to revisit this checklist as needed, as well as others you will find in the next chapters.

- ❏ What is your DTx organization's primary purpose and objective (a.k.a. its "true north")?
- ❏ Who are the most influential stakeholders in your ecosystem (i.e., patients, physicians, partners, or payers)?
- ❏ What are the jobs each of these stakeholder groups is trying to get done?
- ❏ Who are your target users, purchasers, and influencers?
- ❏ What is your systematic, repeatable approach to analyzing stakeholder needs?
- ❏ How do you deliver exceptional utility along the care continuum?
- ❏ How will your organization deliver annual revenues by a targeted time frame?

You should be able to answer all of these questions once you have a clear view of the problem your DTx technology aims to address. A problem well defined is a problem half-solved, right? Using your problem definition as your true north during every stage and pivoting along your organization's strategy is the most direct way to success. All too often, though, developers and entrepreneurs operate in reverse: *they have a solution looking for a problem*, obviating whether the solution is actually needed. Indeed, the absence of a clearly defined market need has always been one of the main drivers of startup failure in any industry, not just in health care.[2]

Our interviews with entrepreneurial health care academics and physicians have yielded key barriers to innovation success. For example, it was noted that health care innovators tend to underestimate early on how a pipeline program and its objectives may adversely impact the viability and scalability of their technology and organization later on. They recognized that major curveballs can often come from erroneous assumptions or insufficiently thought-through ideas about the business model (e.g., direct-to-consumer approach or not), the regulatory perspective (e.g., requirements for regulatory clearance), or the reimbursement pathway. These outcomes can be particularly unfortunate when the technology would in fact be transformative had it been deployed optimally.

The initial steps of forming a DTx organization are indeed critical. Many health technology success stories start with insights from health care professionals, patients, and caregivers to understand their challenges and what potential solutions may look like from their points of view. Even if physicians or patients don't know what they want, cannot visualize what they want, or want a solution for a very specific unmet clinical need that is not addressable at scale—that information contributes to the broader context of your idea's fit. Where applicable and accessible, perspectives from providers, insurers, and other key stakeholders may be vital resources for successful emergence out of the ideation stage.

So the absence of a well-defined market need is a top reason why startups fail, but running out of cash or not having the right team in place are also critical risks. To address these challenges, DTx developers need to identify the right problem across three dimensions (see figure). We will explore each of these dimensions in the following

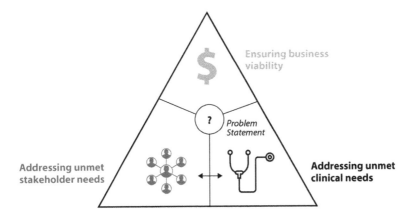

FIGURE PART II.1. Identification of the (right) problem. Source: From the authors

chapters and offer perspectives, tools, and best practices that will help make your venture formation and technology development road map a success. These suggestions further aim to help innovators systematically approach roadblocks, ensuring they are asking the right questions at the outset, and ultimately derisking every step of DTx development.

NOTES
1. Humphreys, "Checklists Save Lives."
2. CB Insights, "The Top 12 Reasons Startups Fail."

CHAPTER 2

Addressing Unmet Stakeholder Needs

This chapter was written with contributions by Fabien Souillard, a patient in France living with type 1 diabetes; Dr. Ester Yeoh, senior consultant at the Diabetes Centre, Admiralty Medical Centre and Division of Endocrinology at Khoo Teck Puat Hospital in Singapore; and Dr. Raj Kumar, certified Blue Ocean Strategy practitioner and CEO of UCSI Blue Ocean Strategy Consulting in Malaysia. Their perspectives are reflected in this chapter to guide you through the exercise of identifying the right problems to solve with DTx.

Fabien was diagnosed with type 1 diabetes when he was 13 years old. The concern that something was wrong started when he began to feel frequently tired and was constantly thirsty. As a result, he began to refuse to go outside his house to play with friends. His family became increasingly worried and were prompted to bring him to the hospital, where the diagnosis was made. At first Fabien didn't comprehend fully what it all meant and how it would impact his lifestyle, but from that point on his life changed. He was started on daily insulin injections and studied how to monitor his blood glucose and carbohydrate intake. Ten years later, after countless consultations with endocrinologists and other physicians, and after countless visits to the hospital to manage his double-digit hemoglobin A1c (HbA1c), stomach cramps, and other complications arising from his condition, he still struggles with daily finger pricks, carbohydrate counting, and trying his best to have the semblance of a "normal" life. Like most people with diabetes, Fabien has not asked for much. He has simply wanted to feel better while minimizing the effort he must put into managing his condition.

Until recently, Fabien had never heard about Omada Health, BlueStar®, or any other diabetes-related DTx platform or app. Moreover, the first time diabetes patients like him were on the verge of experiencing a revolution in their diabetes management was in 2006 when the first inhaled insulin—Exubera—was approved by the FDA. Exubera was a dry powder form of rapid-acting insulin delivered by oral inhalation and labeled (which in regulatory language specifies an approval for a specific condition) for controlling hyperglycemia in adults with type 1 or type 2 diabetes. According to Pfizer, which developed the formulation, Exubera was a major medical and technological breakthrough that promised to replace bothersome insulin injections.

It turned out, however, that not many patients and physicians were interested in using Exubera. After more than a year on the market, despite heavy advertising, Exubera only managed to capture 1% of the insulin market. For this reason, Pfizer ended its production in late 2007 and took a $2.8 billion pretax hit on the product. "Despite our best efforts, Exubera has failed to gain the acceptance of patients and physicians," acknowledged Pfizer's CEO at the time.[1] All things considered, Exubera highlighted the importance of understanding how patients, physicians, and payers approached diabetes management.

From a patient's perspective, the product was challenging to use discreetly, as it was administered through an inhaler about the size of a can of tennis balls. Patients who were willing to use Exubera daily were required to check their lung function at regular intervals as a safety measure. Also, it did not provide an easy way to convert a patient's normal insulin amount into an Exubera-calibrated dosage, leading to concerns about potential dosing errors. As a result, it created considerable operational hurdles and complexities for patients, but also for physicians and the system.

From a physician's perspective, implementation was challenging. Substantial effort was required to educate patients on how to use the Exubera inhaler adequately—a deal-breaker for many physicians considering the limited consultation time available in a busy practice. For instance, in the United Kingdom a general practitioner spends an average of 9.2 minutes with a patient, which is clearly insufficient for any pedagogical activities in addition to the clinical consultation.[2] Also, Exubera did not sufficiently address the issue of conventional insulin administration, as most type 1 patients and a portion of type 2 patients still needed long-acting insulins for basal control of blood sugars.

From a payer's perspective, looking particularly at the cost-effectiveness, the device was 30% more expensive than traditional solutions. *Bloomberg* at the time concluded that "perhaps next time Pfizer will do a little more homework to determine whether an innovative idea truly has a market."[3]

The example of Exubera, a well-known case study in the industry, reminds us that (1) the path from research and development to commercialization is anything but straightforward, and (2) obtaining an FDA approval does not guarantee market adoption. Yet too many organizations and entrepreneurs focus solely on their technology instead of the problem it aims to solve. This condition is referred to sometimes as entrepreneurial myopia, which is when companies are more focused on their product than the needs and requirements of customers.

In the case of Exubera, understanding the problems faced by patients like Fabien, physicians, and other stakeholders involved directly or indirectly in the care of people with diabetes may have prevented entrepreneurial myopia, or corporate myopia. More broadly, prevention should start with diagnosing a potential technological solution's ecosystem—which is typically dynamic and complex in health care—and its direct and indirect stakeholders (figure 2.1), all of whom

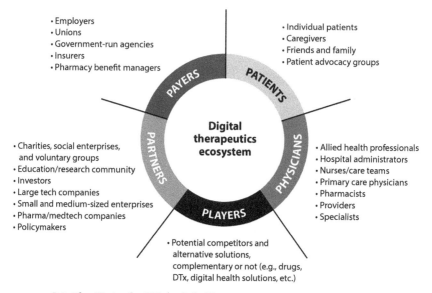

Employers
• Unions
• Government-run agencies
• Insurers
• Pharmacy benefit managers

• Individual patients
• Caregivers
• Friends and family
• Patient advocacy groups

PAYERS

PATIENTS

Digital
therapeutics
ecosystem

• Charities, social enterprises,
  and voluntary groups
• Education/research community
• Investors
• Large tech companies
• Small and medium-sized enterprises
• Pharma/medtech companies
• Policymakers

PARTNERS

PHYSICIANS

• Allied health professionals
• Hospital administrators
• Nurses/care teams
• Primary care physicians
• Pharmacists
• Providers
• Specialists

PLAYERS

• Potential competitors and
  alternative solutions,
  complementary or not (e.g., drugs,
  DTx, digital health solutions, etc.)

FIGURE 2.1. The 5Ps in the DTx stakeholder ecosystem. Source: From the authors

have different roles and objectives. With the rapidly evolving ecosystem at the intersection of health care and technology, DTx teams must be much more externally focused than any other organization and not overlook the needs and goals of any stakeholder group, as they could later turn out to be key catalysts for entrepreneurial success as well as impact to the patient and health care system.

There are numerous ways to slice and dice the stakeholder ecosystem to gain a deeper understanding of how the different agents interact and depend on each other. Key factors for these stakeholders to consider when assessing a pending ecosystem include, but are not limited to,

- evaluating each stakeholder's potential impact;
- understanding their awareness about and interest in adopting DTx solutions;
- the stakeholders' level of influence over others who might adopt the solution; and
- the ability of DTx innovators to influence these stakeholders.

To use a health care analogy, performing a diagnostic analysis of the DTx stakeholder ecosystem should be as thorough as a patient's first consultation with a specialist. These first consultations are typically longer and more extensive as specialists take the time to understand the patient's medical story, check their medical records, understand what matters most to them (oftentimes patients value better functional health more than mere improvement of clinical indicators), and determine how they can help. Similarly, we are suggesting that serious DTx entrepreneurs should begin by conducting a thorough examination and diagnosis of the ecosystem they aim to impact. Doing so goes beyond traditional stakeholder mapping and extends to understanding the challenges and priorities of patients, physicians, and other end users along the care continuum relevant to their specific technology, from disease prevention to diagnosis and management. In the process, they will likely discover that success looks very different to each of these stakeholders and their needs could sometimes be conflicting, which is why it is important to take stock of all these inputs before designing or trying to implement anything.

DTx has the capacity to transform the way that medicine is practiced if solutions are developed and implemented the right way. While a whole-of-community approach among stakeholders to collaborate and address this new frontier is underway, a historical view of health care innovation and the realization of established adoption strategies offer valuable pointers to those seeking to disrupt the field of medicine. For this reason, in this chapter we offer a deep dive into diabetes as a practical exercise of ecosystem diagnosis, sharing the perspectives of Fabien, who has lived with diabetes for more than half his life, and Dr. Ester Yeoh, a physician who recognizes the challenges faced by the myriad of patients from all walks of life that she manages in the clinic.

Fabien and Dr. Yeoh's stories may be unique, but they do have facets of similarity to other stakeholders in the health care ecosystem. Both of them would benefit from a potential DTx solution, either coming from the angle of the person with diabetes or the physician managing that person. Ideally, a DTx solution would be able to satisfy both needs.

Understanding their perspectives on managing diabetes and looking at their current approaches to technology adoption will provide insights into how DTx solutions can fit within their respective routines. In the journey to creating a DTx solution, too, these perspectives will need to be referenced every now and then to ensure that the focus on the end user is not lost. Let's start with looking at the challenges faced by people living with diabetes. With these challenges comes the opportunity for the ideation of effective and adoptable DTx solutions.

Challenges Faced by People Living with Diabetes
Delay in Diagnosis

Diagnosing diabetes is relatively simple in theory. Depending on country-specific guidelines, a single blood test—either an HbA1c test, a fasting plasma glucose test, or an oral glucose tolerance test—could confirm a diagnosis. Singapore is frequently cited as having one of the most efficient health care systems worldwide.[4] Nonetheless, 50% of diabetes cases in Singapore remain undiagnosed, mirroring global estimates of 45.8% undiagnosed, ranging from 24.1% to 75.1% across geographical regions.[5] Increasing awareness of screening locations, improving access to and compliance with clinician follow-up appointments, and harnessing technology are just a few of the many ways to address this issue.[6] Diabetes, including its diagnosis, is a global problem of pandemic proportions, posing challenges to even the most well-funded and efficient health care systems.[7] It is imperative to overcome this barrier to diagnosis because diabetes tends to be the starting point for many other health complications, and if not properly diagnosed and managed, it can lead to cardiovascular, vision, renal, neurological, gastrointestinal, and oral health disorders, to name just a few. In a nutshell, its impact on patient quality of life can be pervasively devastating.

Lack of Awareness and Short-Term Results

Public health messages about diabetes have been widely featured on media channels as well as subway and bus stations ever since Singapore initiated its war on diabetes campaign. However, there remains a segment of the population that lacks awareness of the symptoms of diabetes as well as the burdens of diabetes on everyday life due to the additional daily tasks required to manage this condition. Once this reality sets in, subsequent challenges in keeping diabetes under control quickly becomes a top-of-mind concern for patients, overriding most other priorities. Fabien says, "Injection, diet, exercise . . . it is like brushing your teeth. It's about eating healthy, exercise, medication, you have no break. You need to be cautious all the time. It's particularly frustrating when you think you have done everything right and your blood sugar is still high. It takes a lot to stay under control."

From a patient's perspective, despite the effort required, the reward for the work put into effectively managing diabetes could simply be the absence of symptoms or the absence of complications (such as hypoglycemia, which is low blood sugar as a result of pharmacological therapy for diabetes).[8] Yet the "punishment" for managing it poorly can appear minimal at first; serious complications tend to materialize over time and are thus often underestimated in the present. This can be particularly apparent for younger diabetes patients, who often have an invincible mindset, limiting their ability to assess risks and future consequences.[9] Fabien and his family were frustrated with the constant need to be vigilant without seeing payback for their efforts, so they began to look for more tangible, short-term results that would motivate him to adhere to his treatment routine. "It's more about how I look now than about worrying about a potential kidney problem I might have in ten years," he says. The daily struggle to keep his blood sugar and other indicators in check was resulting in an emotional roller coaster for him. In disease management speak, it was resulting in inconsistent motivation and poor engagement.

For Fabien, it was necessary to start taking insulin immediately after the diagnosis of type 1 diabetes. For people with type 2 diabetes, though, insulin intake usually starts when controlling the disease cannot be achieved with diet, exercise, and oral medications alone. When a person with type 2 diabetes reaches that stage, they may view it as a sign of failure, which is a common misconception.[10] Furthermore, a successful initiation of insulin therapy may be challenging due to medication avoidance from the fear of self-injection and perceived social stigma.

Financial Burden

Individuals with diabetes tend to cover a substantial amount of out-of-pocket costs, which can range from US$143 to US$2,210 per year.[11] These costs include payment for consultations, medications that may include insulin and insulin delivery devices such as insulin pumps, and blood glucose monitoring equipment such as testing strips or glucose sensors. These costs can impede or even preclude access to treatment, which can subsequently lead to suboptimal patient outcomes.

The financial burden of diabetes extends beyond direct health care costs, too. Indirect costs such as those caused by increased absenteeism, reduced productivity at work, or inability to work as a result of a disease-related disability add to the burden, both for the person with diabetes and for society at large.

Challenges Faced by Physicians Caring for Patients with Diabetes

In order to make fully informed decisions when it comes to therapy options, potential referrals, and counseling, physicians need to acknowledge the full spectrum of challenges that lead to suboptimal health outcomes for their patients. Yet, they also have challenges of their own when it comes to supporting people with diabetes.

Time

Time is a major constraint for Dr. Yeoh and for all the health care practitioners we interviewed for this book, be it specialists, general practitioners, or nurses. All mentioned how they wished they could have more time with their patients during consultations so as to fully understand their situations, needs, and potential obstacles to treatment. They all highlighted that a one-size-fits-all approach does not work for people with diabetes because each patient is affected by it in different ways. Importantly, their expectations from the treatment results also vary substantially. Therapeutic options need to be individually tailored and collaboratively arriving at a joint decision requires time.

Diabetes management at a physician's office is a multifaceted process. The physician needs to look through blood glucose records and modify pharmacotherapy while also managing all risk factors simultaneously. This includes monitoring blood pressure, cholesterol levels, cardiovascular risk, smoking history, mental well-being, and more. The physician also ensures and coordinates screening for diabetes complications of the eyes, feet, nerves, and blood vessels as well as any additional problems that may surface during each consultation. It may not be possible for a single consultation to encompass everything that requires discussion, much less follow up on particulars like blood glucose monitoring records. This results in additional out-of-clinic consultations through emails, phone calls, and other modes of contact. These complex processes have even been considered as factors disrupting work-life balance, potentially increasing the risk of physician burnout.

Low Uptake of Diabetes Self-Management Education

Across the landscape of diabetes management, Dr. Yeoh is most passionate about empowering her patients to take charge of their conditions through self-management education. Most health care practitioners and clinics that care for diabetes patients, however, do not receive additional reimbursement for time spent providing nonclinical services. This misalignment of incentives in health care is neither new nor unique to the therapy area of diabetes and is sometimes referred to as "unfavorable economics."

Adding to the time constraint on the provider's end, having diabetes patients come for regularly scheduled educational sessions requires effort and perseverance. The sign-up rates for such programs generally tend to be low and dropouts can reach up to 50%, increasing with each additional day in the program. The reason for these poor attendance numbers is that most patients cannot easily take time off from work or school to attend activities that do not appear to be strictly related to clinical management of their condition, in contrast to the blood sugar, eye, and foot screenings for which they already commit substantial time. Dr. Yeoh has tried to work around those limitations by organizing weekend and online classes but concluded that it's an uphill battle to convince patients to show up consistently when they may not prioritize it themselves.

Confirming Dr. Yeoh's observations, a team of researchers in 2017 investigated factors influencing uptake of structured diabetes self-management education (DSME) by people with type 1 diabetes in order to understand why only about 27% of these patients participated in a common program known as the Dose Adjustment for Normal Eating program.[12] They found associations between attendance at structured education and young age, female gender, and higher HbA1c level (i.e., >75 mmol/mol doubled the chance of attendance). Also, participants from areas of social deprivation[13] were half as likely to attend.

In 2019, these researchers were part of a team that identified five key barriers for attending DSME: psychological capability (the most influential factor), numerical capability (defined as a person's ability to deal with numerical information, particularly in relation to their diabetes self-care), internal/external judgment, thirst for knowledge, and self-confidence.[14] These themes led to the identification of distinct profiles (also referred as "personas") of people with type 1 diabetes with low DSME attendance. This stratification approach can be leveraged by physicians, designers of patient education programs, and DTx developers to define targeted interventions for specific patient subgroups, as the researchers noted. Could there be a DTx solution that enables diabetes education to be brought to the patient seamlessly while incentivizing the patient toward diabetes self-management?

Therapy Nonadherence

Despite a physician's best efforts, people with diabetes may not consistently follow their advice. Therapy nonadherence encompasses skipping prescribed medication, forgoing necessary testing, and not making recommended lifestyle changes. It is estimated that approximately 50% of patients do not take medications as prescribed.[15] The Diabetes Attitudes, Wishes, and Needs Study in 2001 showed that adherence among type 2 diabetes patients was at 78% for medications, 64% for self-monitoring of blood glucose, 37% for diet, and 35% for exercise.[16] There is a high correlation between nonadherence and low socioeconomic status, low education levels, being a member of an ethnic minority, and depression, pointing to issues of inequality and inequity in diabetes management. Importantly, these are also factors to consider in the context of DTx development.

The reported average adherence to long-term chronic illness therapy in developed countries is 50%, implying a similar percentage for nonadherence, according to the World Health Organization.[17] It's reported that about 40% to 50% of diabetes patients in the United States abandon treatment during insulin initiation or intensification, a percentage that can go as high as 70% to 80% in self-pay markets such as India. In all cases, abandoning diabetes treatment contributes to worse health outcomes.[18]

We know that therapy adherence is a key determinant of the effectiveness of a treatment, but it can also have a positive economic impact.[19] In one example, the estimated cost savings of the US health care system associated with improving medication adherence for diabetes patients ranged from $661 million to $1.16 billion.[20]

Therapy nonadherence can be explained in many ways: inconvenience, a low sense of urgency if symptoms are not immediately noticeable or worrisome, low or no awareness about why behavioral change matters, low perception of the risks of nonadherence and the benefits of adherence, and a lack of immediate feedback to patients who do comply with their treatment regimen regarding measurable progress. In a nutshell, for people with diabetes, there is no apparent timely positive return on investment for their personal expense and efforts.

Behavioral Change

The insights from patient and physician have raised a clear point: Behavioral change is at the foundation of a strong arsenal against diabetes.

Instead of viewing diabetes as a constant battle with wins and losses, Fabien has learned to live with it. Ideally, he wants to feel well without his condition overwhelming his daily routines or requiring drastic changes to his lifestyle. Unfortunately, standard treatment requires substantial effort on the part of the patient. This reality is unlikely to satisfy his needs and his personal diabetes goals, resulting in a mismatch of expectations between physician and patient. All things considered, the decisive factor is still Fabien's commitment to adhering to his treatment plan. Those living with type 1 and type 2 diabetes share this struggle.

Numerous studies have defined and assessed different behavior change techniques, but identifying which specific techniques or combinations thereof are potentially effective for a given individual and selected behavior presents a major challenge because behavior itself is not a constant.[21] A patient on Monday morning may be physiologically different, feeling and acting differently, than the same patient on Friday evening. Dynamically managing patient care at scale, then, is currently an enormous challenge, even though studies show that there is a clear correlation between patient behavior change and clinical outcomes, particularly in diabetes.[22]

Complex is probably the word that best encapsulates Fabien's and Dr. Yeoh's experiences in managing diabetes and dealing with its associated challenges of awareness, access to treatment, cost, time, and motivation. Those factors highlight that the difficulties of managing the disease arise not only from its clinical dimensions, but also from the human dynamics around them: the patients, families, caregivers, and health care professionals involved in the direct care of diabetes, as well as the individuals and institutions who have an indirect impact, including public and private payers, employers, technology innovators, and clinician-entrepreneurs who recognize the need for better therapy adherence design. In the context of DTx, the objective is to improve Fabien's quality of life with a seemingly effortless management plan. As for Dr. Yeoh, the objective is to improve glycemic control and lowering glycemic variability to realize positive clinical outcomes while ultimately meeting a patient's expectations and definitions of success.

Pointer

For a 360° view of the DTx ecosystem, including perspectives other than those of patients and clinicians, consider also understanding the perspectives of new groups of relevant stakeholders, such as health care administrators, policymakers (e.g., government and local authorities), payers (e.g., health system organizations, employers, and insurers), academic researchers, investors, or industry players (e.g., biopharmaceutical and medtech organizations).

Different stakeholders have unique views of how successful disease management is defined (table 2.1). Their needs and interests could sometimes conflict. Understanding their priorities, challenges, and how they might be impacted is therefore critical to developing potential solutions. For a systematic, repeatable approach to analyzing stakeholder needs, we detail in the next section of this chapter a theory of consumer action, describing the mechanisms that lead market participants (in our case, health care stakeholders) to adopt an innovation.

Table 2.1. Illustration of key patient and clinician definitions of success and challenges using a DTx lens

	Defining success in the context of DTx	Potential challenges
Patients (plus caregivers or family members of patients)	• Feeling better and having fewer symptoms as a result of DTx-mediated intervention. • Spending less time on managing one's condition while having access to continuous, real-time, digitally generated feedback about current health status. • Navigating and operating the DTx with ease (e.g., simple to access; easy to use in-app charts, graphs, and other pictorial displays). • Experiencing less financial burden.	• Being overwhelmed by an overabundance of apps and solutions available on the market, and knowing how to choose the right one. • Feeling digitally illiterate (a frequent concern for older users) • Inaccessible infrastructure for large segments of the population. • Concern about data protection and privacy.
Clinicians	• Empowering and supporting patients to adopt healthier lifestyles likely to lead to improved outcomes (e.g., improving patient awareness about their condition and the importance of therapy adherence). • Access to digitally generated intermediate outcomes feedback to aid with patient management. • Efficient patient onboarding with a treatment plan. • Augmenting care delivered outside the clinic by adding digitally enabled touchpoints without investing additional effort or time. • Engaging the DTx with ease (e.g., simple to access; easy to use and understand in-app charts, graphs, and other pictorial displays).	• Lacking robust evidence of the DTx's effectiveness (e.g., What are the proven clinical benefits? Can DTx really change patient behavior?). • Adding overhead and ending up spending too much time on nonclinical aspects of care. • Siloed implementation of existing technological solutions, which could impede clinical workflow. • Concern about accountability (Who is to blame if the DTx provides the wrong advice?) • Concern about data protection and privacy. • Lacking access to the appropriate reimbursement models.

Did You Know?

In the last eight minutes you were reading this book, the US government has spent close to $5 million ($4,977,169 to be exact) on diabetes alone, and this is only for patients who have been diagnosed.[23] We will see in the next few chapters how DTx can contribute to having more informed, engaged, and motivated patients for better clinical and financial outcomes.

Defining the Jobs Stakeholders Want to Get Done

Correctly identifying customer or stakeholder priorities and staying focused on them when developing a new product or service is essential to the success of any business, including a DTx startup. Here we offer a systematic approach to understanding stakeholder priorities and unmet needs by using the jobs-to-be-done (JTBD) framework.

In essence, we are all trying to get a job done. When we buy a product, we "hire" it to help us do a job, as described by the theory's author, the late Clayton M. Christensen, who is widely regarded as one of the foremost experts on business growth and disruptive innovation.[24] In this line of reasoning, you may use a drill (product) not to make a hole in the wall, but to hang a frame (job). Similarly, you may buy the latest Bluetooth headset (product) not to listen to music, but to motivate yourself and set your pace when you go running (job).

In our collective experience, we have often seen the difficulties patients, families, and physicians have in clearly articulating their needs. This puts an onus on you, the DTx innovator and creative problem-solver, to figure out what would deliver value (defined differently to each stakeholder) to the collective "them" (which requires a multifaceted vision). Henry Ford, founder of the Ford Motor Company, is known for having famously said, "If I had asked people what they wanted, they would have said faster horses." DTx developers can borrow a page from Ford's book and apply an outcome-focused lens to overcome the challenge of vaguely framed problem definitions. The JTBD framework creates a unique value proposition for each stakeholder in the ecosystem, so they can "get the job done." Simply put, it's ensuring that your future solution will address a real problem.

Adapted from the literature, a JTBD analysis is generally structured as follows:

[Person] wants to [Solve a Problem] in this [Context], so he/she can [Expected Outcomes[25]]

Let's see now how this works by applying it to Fabien's case, our young protagonist with type 1 diabetes. Fabien was growing impatient with the lack of instant feedback or positive reinforcement offered by conventional disease management programs. A DTx entrepreneur might start by applying the JTBD framework to understand why and how Fabien does what he does and the problems he faces that motivate him to buy and use a product. The aim is to understand Fabien's priorities in a particular set of circumstances, the events or situations that trigger a reaction in him, his desired progress, and his motivation for achieving that desired state. For example:

Potential Job #1:
Fabien wants to know what to do (e.g., exercise, monitor his blood glucose, or other indicators, etc.) and what to eat when he is at home alone so he can be confident that he is robustly managing his condition.

This first JTBD definition can lead to a solution, digital or not, that aims to minimize the burden of self-management by simplifying the treatment regimen (e.g., by delivering brief educational "nuggets" on how to prevent blood sugar spikes). For Fabien to feel more empowered, such a solution may take on many forms. Examples include digitally delivered continuous feedback that gives him visibility into how he's doing in terms of therapy adherence, and perhaps positive reinforcement when he's hitting all his goals. Obviously, the solution need not be delivered only during Fabien's regular outpatient visits to the hospital. They can also follow him home, allowing him to stay connected, see tangible results (and reasons) for him to be compliant, and maybe even share his progress with friends or online peers to enable community-driven adherence modalities.

Now notice how this next example can lead to a different, more clinically focused solution:

Potential Job #2:
Fabien wants to feel less bogged down by managing his type 1 diabetes so he can have more time to do fun activities with his friends and family.

This second JTBD definition has to do with therapy optimization and insulin titration, possibly facilitated remotely by a health care provider. It could materialize as a DTx solution that sends an alert to Fabien's treating physician to inform them if it seems like a consultation with a psychologist might benefit the patient at a particular point in time, or if another kind of coaching or motivational program might help with symptom management.

From our experience with designing new products that patients want, there are five sets of questions that should guide this JTBD discovery process:

1. What kind of problem is the patient trying to solve and in what specific circumstance are they trying to solve it?
2. Is there an important problem they have that lacks an adequate solution?
3. How is the patient getting the job done now? What are their compensating behaviors in the absence of an optimal solution?
4. What functional, social, and emotional criteria will the patient use to evaluate whether a potential solution is right for them? Conversely, what functional, social, or emotional factors would take a potential solution "off the table" for them?
5. How would "value" be measured from the patient's perspective?

We asked Fabien to share his perspective on each of these questions. Please remember that Fabien's story is as unique as any other patient's story, and we are not pretending that by understanding him better you will be able to design the right DTx solution for all people with type 1 diabetes. The overarching objective is to instead understand the process and tools that you will need along this discovery journey. Understanding your individual patient's condition—their day-to-day life, activities, and care management as well as therapy needs, options, and challenges—should be the starting point of designing a potential DTx solution. What problem(s) are you trying to solve for your patient? Learning to interpret your patient's frustrations and potential unmet needs (as well as those for every other stakeholder in their ecosystem) and converting them into a neatly defined job to be done is a critical skill. It is not an easy task, but these questions are a good starting point.

What kind of problem are you trying to solve and in what specific circumstance are you trying to solve it?

Fabien: *The long-term side effects of years of uncontrolled diabetes have started to manifest as oral health problems and, more recently, diabetic neuropathy—a type of nerve damage, according to my physician. Coming back to more acceptable glycemic levels is my top priority. In fact, it has always been. I must be successful at managing my diet, exercise, regularly checking my blood sugars, and giving my insulin while maintaining an active life-style* [remember he is only 25 years old] *without having access to solutions that have been proven to be effective for me or other patients, such as the pump.*[26]

From this extract of our discussion with Fabien, his glycemic variability is clearly a short-term problem he is trying to solve. But if you will be having this discussion in the future with a patient community, more patient-provided specifics will be needed to better understand the context and the reasons why, when, and how it is easier (or not) to manage their blood sugar.

Is there an important problem that lacks an adequate solution?

Fabien: *The main problem for me is the relationship with physicians. They know well the theory, the disease evolution and manifestation. I even had endocrinologists who themselves had diabetes, but each patient is different. I know myself. When I have hypos* [low blood glucose], *I know the best ways to get my blood sugar back up quickly without getting hyperglycemia. Many times I can predict my glycemic level without testing myself. However, my physicians are not listening to me enough. My day-to-day experiences are different. I can't stick to a routine and have the same glycemic intake every day, or the same level of physical activity and be in the same emotional state without getting sick.*

How are you getting the job done now? What are your compensating behaviors in the absence of an optimal solution?

Fabien: *I need to test myself more, and I find my ways of doing it by creating my own habits. For example, I have associated each glycemic test with a specific moment of my day so I don't forget. My blood sugar reader is, for example, always near my alarm clock, so it's the first thing I do every morning before snoozing the alarm. I also tend to have a tea break around four p.m. While the coffee gets ready, I do a test, etc.*

For Fabien, these are critical moments of the day where he is constantly reminded of the need to take a test or simply take care of himself. Understanding these moments, which are unique to each patient, is an opportunity to send the right notification or nudge at the right time—which we will explore in more detail later.

Despite established routines and reminders to comply with diabetes management protocols, missed steps are a common reality when living with diabetes. This is where compensatory behaviors come in. Compensatory behaviors are actions patients take to make up for something they should have done—behaviors meant to compensate for something else, a workaround. Fabien knows he is not going to test himself as much as his physician has requested, so he focuses on his food intake and has learned over time how to listen to his body—which is not a perfect solution. Patients with long-standing diabetes may start to lose some of the warning signs of low blood sugar (hypoglycemia) or lose the ability to predict when they are having a hypoglycemic episode, which in turn can result in a more severe episode. Therefore, solutions that provide actionable blood glucose readings without Fabien consciously having to check would be welcome and eliminate the guesswork.

What functional, social, and emotional criteria do you use to evaluate what is right for you? Conversely, what functional, social, or emotional factors would take a potential solution "off the table" for you?

Fabien: *I was initially against the insulin pump. Then I considered what I would gain and found that it promised much more flexibility for meals (partly* emotional and partly social criteria), and I was able to reduce the items I needed to carry around (functional). These advantages outweighed the challenges that would come with it, such as the constant reminder of being sick with diabetes (emotional) or how others would perceive me if I had this device on me all the time (social). A pump would have also been "off the table," as you said, if the potential pain during the initial set-up or during daily usage, or the potential risks such as the risk of infection at the infusion site, outweighed the overall benefits.

How is "value" measured from your perspective?
Fabien: *Value for me, is simply the ratio of benefit and loss for any solution, including the financial aspects and potential co-payment. Not to mention, if you add the patient's willingness to be at the center of his pathology, a convinced patient would probably benefit more from any solution.*

Fabien is looking at value in the form of a yes-no decision when accepting a solution, such as the pump in this example. The value is also related to the notion of success for him, that is, how he defines success and how the value of a solution throughout the evolution of his condition, in one way or the other, will help him feel successful.

When conducting such interviews with patients like Fabien, there are important shortcuts and pitfalls to avoid. In our experience of using the JTBD approach ourselves, we strongly feel that it is equally important to listen to what a patient says *and* observe what he does. Trusting action over statements tends to be a reliable approach to identifying the underlying needs, which is often the limitation of traditional survey-based market research.

We have also realized through patient interviews that it's important to not fall victim to the curse of knowledge in order to avoid cognitive bias. If you know that you are going to interview "Fabien, type 1 diabetes, 25 years old," then there may be preconceived notions and expectations about his challenges and struggles. For this reason, we should focus on the circumstances of the stakeholder rather than their demographic profile. We should look deeper into patterns, themes, and insights to identify the root causes that are driving their needs to prioritize their JTBD.

As we have seen with Fabien, two jobs can lead to different solutions, so the question of which to prioritize is crucial. When there is more than one possible JTBD, consider their importance from the stakeholder's perspective as well as the stakeholder's satisfaction (or lack thereof) with existing solutions. The larger the gap between the two (e.g., important JTBD but unsatisfied with the status quo), the clearer the target area of a DTx platform. Based on this assessment, targets could be developing a new feature, a new functionality, a new way to use the power of data science, or some other entirely novel solution. In the context of the discussion with Fabien, the JTBD approach provided key insights:

1. He has a clear idea of steps needed to manage his condition. Hence, the importance of the first job definition suggested earlier was not high. Solutions developed to tackle this JTBD may not find Fabien as a user.
2. Achieving the targets of the second job definition is a priority for Fabien. At the same time, current solutions do not satisfy his requirements. Hence, a user-identified target for DTx development or improvement may have emerged.

To conclude, JTBD is one of many approaches available for uncovering the key factors that drive an individual's health behaviors. Regardless of the approach used, it is critical for DTx organizations to perform such analyses as they craft new functionalities to perform better than existing alternatives and at the same time address or leverage current compensating behaviors. Comprehensively considering these points will realize a DTx that fulfill users' functional, social, and emotional needs in a true customer-centric approach.

Addressing Pain Points and Delivering Value to Stakeholders

Now that we've considered the importance of understanding the patient and provider perspective when developing DTx platforms, it's time to think about the aforementioned objective of delivering stakeholder value. Finding a winning business idea entails understanding the pain points of the industry you are working with and, more importantly, of your stakeholders. In health care, this typically means focusing on meeting the needs of and overcoming the challenges confronted by patients, caregivers, and physicians. Established and aspiring DTx innovators can approach this process by systematically analyzing and empathizing with their potential future users, understanding the pain points they experience at every stage of their journey, and figuring out how a DTx solution can help them overcome those barriers and unlock utility or new value (figure 2.2).

Fabien's ideal end-to-end patient journey spans from seeing his specialist, to being offered a new DTx that helps him manage his diabetes, to ultimately a "digital exit," which is achieved when a patient may not need the DTx any longer. This journey can be visually understood by applying W. Chan Kim and Renée Mauborgne's concept of the Buyer Utility Map.[27] According to this concept, Fabien may experience different emotions and pain points during his patient journey. These emotions and pain points can be organized into five categories: productivity, simplicity, convenience, risk reduction, and fun and image. These categories—also called utility levers—help user experience researchers (a role DTx innovators should consider incorporating into their teams) label and group pain points and obstacles in a more systematic and granular way, instead of simply asking a patient "What are the challenges you face in this journey?" and relying on his spontaneous response at that moment.

Applying a systematic approach to the pain point discovery process helps us stay focused on solving the real problem at hand while eliminating the potential myopia of pure novelty, which all too often leads to innovators having that solution still looking for a problem. Rather, DTx entrepreneurs should strive to create demand-driven products instead of supply-driven ones. A systematic analysis of the user journey is imperative in therapeutics in general, but especially so in digital

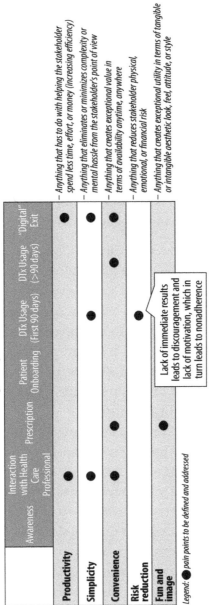

FIGURE 2.2. Pulling the right levers to deliver utility. Source: Adapted from the Buyer Utility Map in Kim and Mauborgne, *Blue Ocean Strategy*; for illustration purposes only

therapeutics, because it provides a simple yet powerful framework to test the desirability of a therapeutic while taking user centeredness into consideration.

Once the pressure points are defined, the solution can be framed around the findings and address each point one by one, as organized by the utility levers. Using this framework in the postmortem analysis of Exubera, Pfizer's rapid-acting inhaled insulin formula, we can begin to appreciate why it failed to unlock exceptional utility for Fabien and other diabetes patients. From a breakthrough novelty standpoint, Exubera seemed to hold great promise because it potentially meant that people with diabetes could move away from the inconvenience and stigma of needle injections. Nevertheless, the shortcomings were evident from a utility point of view.

- *Stakeholder productivity.* Despite the cleverness of the underlying technology, the size of the inhaler was too big and cumbersome to handle. Even for a young person like Fabien, holding it properly posed a challenge. Apart from that, using the product was a time-consuming procedure since it required inserting a series of blisters and activating the pump before the inhaler was ready to be used. Of note, this process took several minutes in contrast to insulin injections, which typically take only a few seconds to administer.
- *Simplicity.* Pfizer underestimated the complexity of using their product, which required selecting a specific insulin dose—a difficult task and major ask for the patient and doctor. Most patients like Fabien would have needed extra education on how to measure and select a dose in order to use the product, which in turn would have required that physicians and nurses spend extra time to educate their patients.
- *Convenience.* The issue of convenience was one of the main reasons for this product's failure—it was not designed with ease-of-use considerations. Its size made it a challenge to carry around and its usage inconvenient.

- *Risk reduction.* The product was priced at a premium, three to four times the average daily cost of injected insulin for a type 1 diabetics.[28] As such, it created a financial risk instead of reducing it. To address this risk, most patients were keen to test the device first before committing to the higher expenditure. Pfizer, however, did not make such an option available. Apart from that, physicians were concerned that it could lead to the development of lung disease in users. In the absence of a long-term clinical trial informing about Exubera's safety and efficacy, it was not recommended to children, smokers, or patients with lung diseases, such as asthma or chronic obstructive pulmonary disease.[29]
- *Fun and image.* This is a utility lever that is often overlooked in the health care industry because of the dominant focus on functionality, yet for some products the emotional proposition is as important as their effectiveness, particularly when it comes to lifestyle integration. In Exubera's case, as previously stated, the product was not discrete, which could lead to unwelcome attention in groups or public. Furthermore, it appears that the inhaler's designers had not given much thought to what would have made Fabien want to show off his new gadget with style and accessories.

Outside of the diabetes arena, a striking example of successfully analyzing and addressing the fun and image lever is in the pediatrics mental disorders field. Akili's EndeavorRx, an FDA-cleared DTx for children with attention deficit hyperactivity disorder (ADHD), is delivered in the form of a video game and its young users are not considered patients or customers by Akili, but "players" who steer a craft through obstacle courses to collect targets (figure 2.3). Gamification, or the use of game design elements, is a unique proposition that can be integrated into DTx to reimagine treatment modalities and boost patient engagement. Playing a computer game to treat a disorder—does this sound too futuristic, or is a reimagination of care delivery in order?

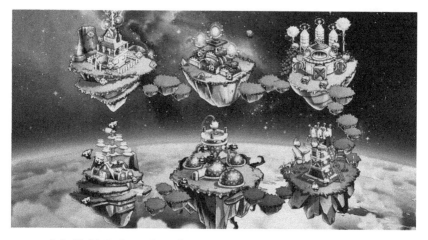

FIGURE 2.3. Akili's EndeavorRx video game interface. Source: Photo by Akili Inc., 2021

Gamification is a promising way to improve patient engagement and disease self-management. By deploying behavioral strategies to unobtrusively motivate users to complete actions, these games may help users stick to their treatment plans more effectively than traditional approaches. That said, gamifying processes requires a focused study and understanding of the solution or product's end users. In Akili's case, they are children and their caregivers.

Applying the concept of utility levers when developing a new DTx product is essential to helping organizations avoid the risk of their offering not gaining traction or failing to be adopted, despite any novelty. Companies that understand the importance of utility levers and design solutions based on this understanding can significantly derisk their operations in solving the right problem and unlocking practice-changing utility to patients, caregivers, and physicians.

Understanding the Buying Decision Process

After running a diagnostic of the ecosystem, understanding the jobs that stakeholders are trying to get done, and figuring out the levers that need to be pulled to deliver exceptional utility, there is one more important consideration that needs to be grappled with: that of understanding the chain of potential buyers for a DTx and knowing where in that chain to focus on. The concept of a "chain of buyers" was introduced by Kim and Mauborgne of Blue Ocean Strategy in 2002.[30] It's a simple yet insightful tool that helps entrepreneurs broaden their vision and narrow their focus at the same time.

The purchase of any product or service involves a chain of people who are directly or indirectly involved in the buying decision. That includes the users of the solution, the purchasers who pay for it, and increasingly often, the influencers whose opinions can make a difference. In Europe, for example, where health services are typically free or near-free at the point of care under a system of universal health coverage, the chain of buyers involved in the decision-making process for starting insulin pump therapy for a patient is strongly influenced by the opinions of endocrinologists and health care providers directly involved in the care of the person with diabetes, such as diabetes nurse educators and dietitians. These professionals are important buyers because they assist patients in analyzing clinical and economic risks, implications, and benefits of the therapy, and patients, mostly, value and trust the opinion of their health care providers. Whether or not a health care provider recommends such a product to the patient is, in turn, influenced by their knowledge of and familiarity with the product, past experience (both positive and negative), and additional factors (such as reliability or responsiveness of technical support, etc.). In contrast, in self-pay markets such as India, the decision-making system for the same therapy is strongly influenced by patients themselves and their families, who generally want to understand the costs of the pumps, supplies, and so on, as well as treatment options presented to them by their health care provider, and compare them with the alternatives of nearby hospitals and providers.

Focusing on and understanding the chain of buyers who might influence a buying decision should be one of a DTx innovator's top priorities as it is an important step in the ecosystem diagnosis and in designing value propositions that address stakeholders' jobs to be done.

Case Study: Medtronic

Medtronic, a leader in medical technology known for its focus on diabetes management, saw in 2011 what the company believed was an untapped market in India—pregnant women with gestational diabetes mellitus (GDM). GDM is a condition in which blood sugar levels become elevated during pregnancy, usually from 24 weeks of gestation onward. While GDM is typically a short-term condition that lasts only for the duration of the pregnancy and shortly thereafter, it increases the risk of type 2 diabetes, a long-term condition. Additionally, GDM can negatively affect healthy development of the baby.[31] India has an especially high rate of GDM, with prevalence ranging from 3.8% to 17.9% of all pregnancies depending on the part of the country.[32] Pregnant women whose GDM is inadequately controlled through dietary measures need to move on to insulin injections or start using insulin pumps.

An insulin pump is an insulin delivery device designed to mimic the way a human pancreas works by delivering small, precise doses of short-acting insulin continuously and other variable amounts of insulin when a meal is eaten. However, an insulin pump in India costs between US$2,500 to US$6,500, amounts which are prohibitive for most Indian women with the need for short-term diabetes control.[33] The cost of the device could effectively be a barrier to treatment for a substantial segment of the population.

Medtronic recognized the underserved market for its insulin pumps in India, where there were about 435,000 women (420,000 pregnant women with GDM as well as 15,000 women with type 1 or 2 diabetes prior to the pregnancy) who were eligible for a pump but were not using one. To address this gap, Medtronic decided to shift its perspective from the influencers (traditionally physicians and endocrinologists)

Table 2.2. Influencer and user concerns regarding insulin pumps for gestational diabetes mellitus (GDM)

Influencers (physicians)	Users (patients)
• Lack of knowledge, familiarity, education, and training on insulin pumps for GDM, leading to limited awareness and knowledge among physicians. • Lack of experience and conviction that insulin pumps are appropriate for managing GDM. • Time-consuming education and hand-holding for patients during the initial introduction to insulin pump therapy. • Relatively high upfront and recurring costs of insulin pumps to patients. • Patients may not turn up for the regular follow-ups that are needed in managing GDM, which requires close monitoring and titration of insulin doses with each trimester.	• Low awareness of the availability of such a technology. • Poor self-testing. • Affordability, high upfront cost, and recurring cost of consumables (e.g., infusion sets and reservoirs/cartridges). There is also concern about what happens to the insulin pump after GDM. • Fear of needles/cannula going under the skin. • The dislike of having a device attached at all times. • Steep initial learning curve to understand how to operate the pump and trouble-shoot in a short time frame.

to the users (GDM and pre–gestational diabetes patients) and focus on understanding their needs and addressing their barriers to treatment (table 2.2).

The Medtronic team quickly identified the device cost as the most commonly stated adoption barrier by not only patients but also by physicians who were reluctant to suggest what was seen as an expensive therapy to their patients. The company thus decided to develop an affordable solution for Indian women with GDM and at the same time work to convince their physicians of the value of insulin pumps for this condition. After experimenting with several business models, Medtronic settled on rolling out a rental program. For about US$150 per month, GDM patients could rent an insulin pump instead of buying one. The company started to test how appealing an insulin pump rental program would be for this group of potential users who were resistant to pay the full cost of the pump upfront. Would they be willing to rent used pumps in the first place? Was the price right?

A shift in the target segment from the influencers to the users revealed a series of unknowns and assumptions that needed to be reevaluated. Medtronic had to not only test how appealing their concept would be to the patients and to the physicians but also assess the overall feasibility of the program from an operational and financial perspective. Would the physicians be willing to prescribe insulin pumps for GDM patients? How intensive would patient training and education need to be? Could Medtronic develop a system to track and distribute the pumps broadly, at scale? What about payment collection? Would the number of GDM patients per hospital or clinic be sufficient to service this program efficiently? The questions were numerous but vital toward establishing the feasibility of this approach.

The two distribution models, purchasing and rental, were offered concurrently. During the pilot program, Medtronic observed that four times more women[34] who rented the insulin pump would ultimately buy their own pump as compared to the women who were not offered the rental program. With this promising result, Medtronic decided to go one step further and integrate this innovative "try before you buy" model into its core business model for servicing type 1 and type 2 diabetes patients. Shifting its focus from the influencers to the users and purchasers allowed Medtronic to not only unlock a new target segment, but also markedly increase the size of its business in India.

The "try before you buy" model, which convinced diabetes patients to sign up for the pump therapy with a relatively small rental fee addressed both the issue of patient affordability as well as the physicians' concerns about suggesting expensive treatment options to their patients. It also achieved a rare feat in health care: giving users an opportunity to try a drug or a medical device before making a long-term commitment. This pilot program has also convinced more physicians to get on board with recommending insulin pumps by increasing the physicians' knowledge and experience with the device.

Testing the assumptions that came with this shift of focus in the chain of buyers was critical to the success of Medtronic's program. It's a powerful example of how to approach a situation where technology alone is not enough to solve a problem, especially in health care.

Medtronic had to question the practicality of its standard commercial model in a different market such as India, invest effort and forward thinking, and be willing to apply what it learned to revamp their business model. In this particular case, the right strategy led to unexpected success that surpassed initial presumptions.

A shift of focus in the chain of buyers is not necessarily a shift from a business-to-business to a business-to-consumer operating model, or to a potentially more complex model. It's also not about new brand positioning. Rather, as the Medtronic example demonstrates, it is about making changes to your business model and unlocking new user research capabilities that you may need to develop or acquire. It also requires addressing stakeholder jobs-to-be-done and potential pain points with which they may be faced, as discussed earlier.

Conclusion

In this chapter we took a closer look at traditional diabetes management to demonstrate the critical importance of assessing stakeholder needs and its impact on the medical and commercial outcomes of a new health care endeavor such as DTx. Commercial use cases demonstrated the different ends of the spectrum that are achievable as a result of addressing these needs. DTx organizations should build on these learnings to successfully develop solutions that can turn invention into innovation, catalyzed by optimally serving the stakeholders involved.

We believe indeed that the most successful organizations are those that solve problems at the intersection of patient and physician jobs-to-be-done and unmet needs, with the solutions also meeting the requirements of stakeholders further downstream. Visionary founders and developers ask questions, listen, and study carefully the challenges key stakeholders face to find and define their intersection because they know that delivering value to both patients and physicians is the way to develop a solution that will be adopted. The patient-physician perspectives outlined in this chapter serve as examples of experiences on the ground, and there are many more stakeholders involved in the health care and DTx ecosystem whose pain points need to be identified and addressed. DTx developers and entrepreneurs should therefore be prepared to build acceptance for the changes that these new technologies will inevitably cause in the broader ecosystem, in addition to developing new technologies. As one of our contributors reminds us,

> We always start with the problems, the inefficiencies we want to address in health care. How we may address these problems may evolve over time and require a few pivots because of our continuous learnings, because our partners may be different, or because of the market-to-market specificities. Regardless of the context, though, for us it's about moving from a transactional to a programmatic way of delivering care and doing so in a more integrated manner to ultimately deliver tangible and proven outcomes.   —Azran Osman-Rani, CEO of Naluri, aspiring DTx company based out of Malaysia that addresses physical and mental health holistically through professional, confidential health coaching.[35]

It's worth repeating: a problem well-defined is a problem half-solved.

NOTES

1. Martino, Hollis, and Teichert, "Pharma's Biggest Flops."
2. Gallagher, "GP Appointments Should Be at Least 15 Minutes in Future."
3. Wientraub, "Pfizer's Exubera Flop."
4. Chen and Wong, "Singapore Beats Hong Kong in Health Efficiency."
5. Singapore Ministry of Health, "National Health Survey 2010"; National Medical Research Council, *Diabetes Taskforce Report.*
6. Institute of Mental Health, "Singapore Residents Show a High Recognition of Diabetes."
7. World Health Organization, "Diabetes: Key Facts."
8. Toh and Wong, "The Big Read: Apathy, Complacency—the Worst Enemies in Singapore's War against Diabetes."
9. King et al., "Perceptions of Adolescent Patients of the 'Lived Experience' of Type 1 Diabetes."
10. American Diabetes Association, "Insulin Myths and Facts."
11. Davis, Burgen, and Chen, "Out-of-Pocket Costs for Patients with Type 2 Diabetes Mellitus."

12. Harris et al., "Factors Influencing Attendance at Structured Education for Type 1 Diabetes in South London"; McIntyre, "Dose Adjustment for Normal Eating: A Role for the Expert Patient?"

13. The English Index of Multiple Deprivation combines information from seven domains to produce an overall relative measure of deprivation. The domains are income, employment, education, skills and training, health and disability, crime, barriers to housing services, and living environment.

14. Harris et al., "Characterization of Adults with Type 1 Diabetes Not Attending Self-Management Education Courses."

15. Brown and Bussell, "Medication Adherence: WHO Cares?"

16. Peyrot et al., "Psychosocial Problems and Barriers to Improved Diabetes Management."

17. World Health Organization, *Adherence to Long-Term Therapies: Evidence for Action.*

18. Riddle, Rosenstock, and Gerich, "The Treat-to-Target Trial: Randomized Addition of Glargine or Human NPH Insulin to Oral Therapy of Type 2 Diabetic Patients."

19. Kennedy-Martin, Boye, and Peng, "Cost of Medication Adherence and Persistence in Type 2 Diabetes Mellitus."

20. Egede et al., "Medication Nonadherence in Diabetes: Longitudinal Effects on Costs and Potential Cost Savings from Improvement."

21. Michie et al., "Evaluating the Effectiveness of Behavior Change Techniques in Health-Related Behavior."

22. Hood et al., "Effective Strategies for Encouraging Behavior Change in People with Diabetes."

23. American Diabetes Association, "The Cost of Diabetes."

24. Christensen et al., "Know Your Customers' 'Jobs to be Done.'"

25. In this context, by "outcomes" we are referring to short-term progress or wins rather than to the clinical outcomes of managing a chronic disease.

26. As per guidance from the National Institute for Health and Care Excellence's *Continuous Subcutaneous Insulin Infusion for the Treatment of Diabetes Mellitus,* "insulin pump therapy is recommended as a treatment option for adults and children 12 years and older with type 1 diabetes mellitus provided that: [1] attempts to achieve target haemoglobin A1c (HbA1c) levels with multiple daily injections (MDIs) result in the person experiencing disabling hypoglycaemia . . . defined as the repeated and unpredictable occurrence of hypoglycaemia that results in persistent anxiety about recurrence and is associated with a significant adverse effect on quality of life, or [2] HbA1c levels have remained high (that is, at 8.5% [69 mmol/mol] or above) on multiple daily injections therapy (including, if appropriate, the use of long-acting insulin analogues) despite a high level of care" (p. 4).

27. Kim and Mauborgne, *Blue Ocean Strategy.*

28. Japsen, "Inhaled Insulin's Cost May Take Breath Away."

29. Barclay, "Exubera Approved Despite Initial Lung Function Concerns."

30. Kim and Mauborgne, *Blue Ocean Strategy*.

31. Wei, "Nurture or Nature? Research Project Reveals Answers."

32. Chudasama et al., "Magnitude of Gestational Diabetes Mellitus."

33. Kesavadev et al., "Use of Insulin Pumps in India: Suggested Guidelines Based on Experience and Cultural Differences."

34. Women with preexisting diabetes and not GDM.

35. From an interview with the authors, June 24, 2020.

CHAPTER 3

Addressing Unmet Clinical Needs

Brian Harris is a board-certified music therapist and one of only 350 people in the world to hold the distinction of Neurologic Music Therapy Fellow.[1] Seeing firsthand the impact of neurologic music therapy (a research-based system of 20 standardized clinical techniques for sensorimotor training, speech and language training, and cognitive training) on his patients at the Spaulding Rehabilitation Hospital in Boston who had suffered such neurologic injuries as stroke, brain injury, or Parkinson's disease, Harris became convinced of its therapeutic value and began searching for a way to expand its impact beyond the rehabilitation hospital. That's how MedRhythms was born in 2015. A neurorehabilitation company Harris cofounded with business entrepreneur Owen McCarthy, MedRhythms focuses on developing and bringing to market DTx solutions that use sensors, music, and software to digitize therapeutic interventions based on the neuroscience research of how music is processed by the brain.

Music has been shown to activate the areas of the brain responsible for movement, language, attention, memory, executive function, and emotion.[2] Thus, the first question MedRhythms had to answer at the start of its DTx endeavor was which of these areas they were to focus on:

We decided to initially focus on walking because of the strong evidence and research in this field. There are over 50 clinical research studies demonstrating improvements in movement when using Rhythmic Auditory Stimulation (RAS). One of those studies showed that each 0.1 meter per second increase in walking speed [as a result of RAS] was correlated to a 7% decrease in fall risk.[3] It was also important to have the ability to measure improvements, such as walking speed and walking quality. The overall objective was functional improvement.

Regarding the indication, there was also strong evidence with trials demonstrating improved walking when RAS was delivered for a rehabilitation after stroke, and in multiple sclerosis (MS), cerebral palsy, and Parkinson's disease. We narrowed the therapeutic areas down to MS, for which there was already a drug on the market, and stroke, where there was a high unmet need with literally no standard-of-care and no solution. In the US alone, there are about 3.5 million chronic stroke patients with walking deficits who have been told they would not be able to walk better again. The cost to the health and social care system is substantial.

—Owen McCarthy, president and cofounder of MedRhythms, member of the Digital Therapeutics Alliance Board of Directors[4]

For any pharmacological, medical, or health technology innovation, choosing a therapeutic area (TA) to focus on is ultimately about addressing unmet clinical needs, a process that begins with a thorough clinical need assessment. For DTx innovators, this means defining and prioritizing the gaps and deficiencies in the current delivery and practice of health care that a potential DTx solution could address. There are many different ways to go about this, but we suggest starting with five fundamental questions that will help you identify the right TA to focus on and guide your reflective process:

1. What are the conditions driving health care utilization?
2. Where is the demand outgrowing health care capacity?

3. What are some underrecognized and undertreated conditions for which a DTx could provide a solution?
4. Who can benefit from behavioral change interventions?
5. What treatment pathways can be improved with a more personalized approach?

Let's do a deep dive into each of these questions.

What Are the Conditions Driving Health Care Utilization?

In a 2008 study exploring the relationship between multimorbidity (concurrent diseases and combinations of diseases a person may have) and use of general practice services in the Dutch population for those 55 years and older, researchers wanted to understand how multimorbidity, which is common among older people, affects the demand for health services. One of the variables they examined, which is seen as a proxy for health care resource utilization, was the number of contacts each of the patients had with a general practice per year (table 3.1). A contact was defined as a face-to-face consultation, a phone contact,

Table 3.1. Total number of contacts with general practice for people with one or more chronic diseases (2014)

Disease	Number of chronic diseases				
	1	2	3	4	≥5
Heart failure	16.7	22.0	26.6	30.0	36.7
Diabetes	14.4	18.5	23.3	26.6	32.3
Chronic obstructive pulmonary disease	13.6	17.2	22.4	25.3	32.1
Stroke	12.9	17.7	21.8	25.1	29.4
Anxiety disorder	12.8	17.6	22.1	25.6	—
Depression	12.7	17.7	23.2	26.8	32.3
Coronary heart disease	11.8	17.1	21.8	25.7	31.7
Cancer	11.5	16.8	21.4	23.1	32.0
Osteoarthritis	10.8	16.2	20.7	23.4	28.4
Chronic back or neck disorder	9.4	14.7	19.2	23.8	27.9

Source: Van Oostrom et al., "Multimorbidity of Chronic Diseases and Health Care Utilization in General Practice."

or a home visit initiated by or on behalf of each patient with one or more chronic diseases.

The mean of the total number of contacts per year was 6.1 for individuals without any chronic diseases (people who can be categorized as "healthy individuals" for simplicity purposes), 11.7 for individuals with a single chronic disease, and 18.3 for individuals with multiple diseases. These statistics confirm what most of us intuitively know: that patients with more chronic conditions tend to need and use more health services. It is interesting to note that in the study, heart failure, diabetes, chronic obstructive pulmonary disease, stroke, anxiety disorder, and depression—in this order—drove the greatest number of contacts for people who had one or more of those conditions. As the researchers noted, a higher number of chronic diseases was associated with more contacts but also with more written prescriptions, and more referrals to specialized care.[5]

The relationship between health conditions that result in high use of health care resources and health system sustainability and efficiency (or inefficiency) is complex and nonlinear. While a discussion of this correlation and its impact on health economics in general is beyond the scope of this book, we would venture that resource-intensive health conditions are a good starting point for DTx innovators. They provide a sound rationale for exploring if and how a DTx can benefit both the patients with these conditions and the broader system by delivering health improvements in a more cost-efficient manner than current treatments and their associated resource requirements do.

It is important to keep in mind that while the conditions mentioned in the study were identified as leading to frequent health care resource utilization in the Dutch health care system, in other countries and geographies the makeup of the costliest diseases may be different. In this broader health care context, however, these figures provide important insight for DTx entrepreneurs to consider where they may have impactful opportunities to develop and implement their solutions.

Where Is the Demand Outgrowing Health Care Capacity?

Resource-intensive diseases are associated with an increased demand for health services that in many places are outgrowing the system's capacity. Globally, nurses and midwives account for nearly 50% of the health workforce and are the backbone of many health care systems,[6] yet they routinely spend precious time performing administrative tasks instead of providing direct care to patients. As a consequence, many of them feel that their time is mismanaged and could be better spent if they were instead allowed to focus on managing, supporting, and educating patients. Taking nurses away from direct patient care and forcing excessive admin work upon them is particularly inadequate when we consider that many health care systems struggle with a shortage of nurses—1,000 people can be attended to by 11.7 nurses in the United States, 9 in countries that are members of the Organisation for Economic Co-operation and Development (OECD), and only 2.7 and 1.7 in China and India, respectively.[7]

The situation with regard to specialists such as ophthalmologists, neurologists, and psychiatrists is similar. The shortage of specialists makes apparent the inequality of access to health care between high-, middle-, and low-income countries. For example, for every 1 million people in the developed markets, there are 76.2 ophthalmologists. In the developing markets this number drops to 3.7 ophthalmologists per 1 million people.[8] With a growing aging population worldwide, the problem of health care resource shortages across therapy areas is only expected to deepen.

Whether you are in a developed or developing market, there is a high chance that you are going to quickly find areas along the care continuum and within specialties where the demand for health care services is outgrowing health care system capabilities. Examining in-depth these areas and whether your potential DTx solution can help alleviate those pressures, could constitute an important element of your value proposition.

What Are Some Underrecognized and Undertreated Conditions for which a DTx Technology Could Provide a Solution?

There are several thousand known diseases that affect humans, but only about 500 of them have treatments approved by the US Food and Drug Administration (FDA).[9] In addition, for some of these diseases, medication can only help control the symptoms and cannot cure the underlying cause. There are more than 6,800 of these diseases affecting an estimated 25 million to 30 million Americans[10] and are typically not financially attractive targets for developing novel pharmacological solutions for because of the small markets each represents individually. While not viable as business opportunities to pharmaceutical companies mainly due to the lengthy, expensive, and high-risk drug development process, rare diseases still account for a huge proportion of the health burden both to patients and their families, and to the health care system at large.[11] They could be a good target for DTx development due to the potential of markedly shorter times to market.

Among the more prevalent conditions for which there is currently no effective treatment, but could be ripe for digital disruption, are Alzheimer's disease and Parkinson's disease. Billions of dollars have been invested in research into potential cures for both, but efforts to develop drugs that effectively treat memory loss and tremor (the primary symptoms of each of those diseases, respectively) have so far been unsuccessful. While a recent FDA approval for an Alzheimer's drug to be used was granted in 2021—the first of its kind in nearly 20 years—promising drugs have repeatedly failed in phase 3 clinical studies.[12] Alzheimer's disease and other dementias contribute to human suffering at scale, and both Alzheimer's and Parkinson's have been listed among the World Health Organization's top 10 diseases that cause the most deaths worldwide.[13]

Another example of underrecognized and undertreated conditions are neurological diseases leading to cognitive impairments, such as schizophrenia, stroke, autism, and traumatic brain injury. Among those, stroke is the main cause of long-term disability. Up to six months after suffering a stroke, two-thirds of survivors have difficulty walking, and beyond six months over 30% still cannot walk without assistance.[14] While individuals with stroke receive rehabilitation training, it rarely lasts more than a few months after reaching a plateau in functional recovery.[15] Often due to a lack of resources for providing long-term services, this is where the science of neuroplasticity, as the basis of an effective DTx solution, could potentially help these patients.

The ultimate goal of stroke care is to recover and maximize the brain functions that have been lost due to cerebral damage. Brain rehabilitation therapy focuses on providing stimulation for neurons to promote brain plasticity—which is the ability of neural wiring to change (e.g., abandon old and form new connections). To further bolster this segment of treatment, digital neurotherapeutics have recently emerged. This subcategory of DTx has the potential to specifically target health deterioration associated with cognitive impairments by targeting the neurological functions that can be remedied with cognitive training. There are various technologies being developed and used in DTx that can deliver "repetitive, goal-oriented tasks with variability while providing performance feedback."[16] To put it more simply, think of the DTx solutions we have discussed so far and their targeted stimulation strategies—for example, Akili Interactive using a video game (see chapter 2) and MedRhythms using music—as a "gym for the brain" that strengthens and expands patients' cognitive capabilities.

Identifying an unaddressed gap to target your DTx requires careful study and understanding of patients' lived experiences with under-recognized and undertreated conditions. For those with conditions for which there is no existing treatment or cure, effective symptom management is still the best option. *This is exactly where DTx can be of greatest value.* We saw an example of this at the beginning of this book in the context of Simon's experience with pain management, where an intelligently designed therapeutic app helped him in ways no pharmacological treatment was able to achieve. Pain management is also a topic of utmost importance to the chronic pain and palliative/hospice care communities, where demand is outgrowing health care capability and capacity. A pain management DTx may offer an opportunity to mimic or replicate to a certain extent the reach of effective pain care to those who cannot avail themselves of it via conventional channels, effectively creating a new care delivery model.

Who Can Benefit from Behavioral Change Interventions?

Following years of research, clinical studies, and practice, cognitive behavioral therapy (CBT) has become a widely used therapeutic approach and is considered a gold-standard in psychotherapy[17] "for a range of problems, including depression, anxiety disorders, alcohol and drug use problems, marital problems, eating disorders, and severe mental illness."[18] Over the years, many traditional cognitive behavioral therapists have also transitioned to digital formats, creating a digital cognitive behavioral therapy (dCBT) category. This is the direction taken by Omada Health, today one of the most highly valued digital health companies.

In 2011, Omada Health decided to "revolutionize health care through group-based programs for chronic disease prevention," and their efforts were initially focused on diabetes.[19] Specifically, the company digitized evidence-based behavioral treatments that were traditionally conducted in clinical face-to-face settings, such as the Centers for Disease Control and Prevention's Diabetes Prevention Recognition Program in the United States. Since then, Omada Health has expanded the digital delivery of behavioral therapy to other indications, too, expanding its programs to address musculoskeletal, prediabetes and weight management, hypertension and behavioral health (i.e., focusing on improving mental health) categories.

This expansion to other conditions represents a common theme at the core of many DTx solutions—the possibility to leverage mechanisms to drive behavioral change aimed at stabilizing, improving, or potentially reversing a condition. Blue Note Therapeutics is also a case in point. They aim to assist cancer patients who commonly experience psychosocial distress, anxiety, or depression.[20] As a result, Blue Note

Therapeutics's solution incorporates cognitive behavioral stress management (CBSM), an evidence-based protocol adapted from CBT and relaxation stress management, designed specifically for patients with cancer. Clinical studies have indeed indicated that CBSM can improve cancer patients' emotional well-being, physical health, and overall survival.[21]

As these real examples demonstrate, DTx platforms are seeking to address an increasing range of diverse medical conditions, such as anxiety disorders, depression, mental health, pain management, allergies, rheumatoid arthritis, gastrointestinal, insomnia, and substance abuse disorders, just to name a few. Behavioral change strategies such as those embedded in DTx leveraging dCBT are also designed to improve therapy adherence—a critical problem across most therapy areas, which has significant clinical and economic implications.

If research into the effectiveness of digital modalities in targeted areas is still being conducted, conditions that can benefit from CBT, and dCBT by extension, would be a good starting point for DTx innovators to consider, and of potential great interest for patients or future patients.[22]

What Treatment Pathways Can Be Improved with a More Personalized Approach?

Since no two patient profiles are alike, health care needs to move beyond the familiar one-size-fits-all models of prevention, diagnosis, and treatment. Following clinical trials, real-world implementation of treatment approaches is confronted with highly diverse patient profiles, and the administration of treatments derived and validated using population-based strategies is too often based on trial and error, with physicians following available guidelines and their own experience. If a particular configuration turns out to be ineffective, the physician proceeds to prescribing a second-line treatment, then a third-line one, and so on until identifying one that works. That is a common pattern that affects a broad spectrum of patients ranging from those with hypertension to cancer. In these scenarios the same therapy may have different results in two patients with the same diagnosis. In fact, even a single patient's response to the same therapy may change over the course of treatment. The shift toward truly personalized care is therefore a particularly important opportunity for DTx.

To try and address this health care challenge, our team at the N.1 Institute for Health at the National University of Singapore has been pioneering N-of-1 (personalized) clinical trials to optimize treatment outcomes at the single-patient level. In 2018, for example, a patient with advanced prostate cancer was provided with a combination of an experimental drug and an approved cancer medication. The patient responded to treatment, demonstrated by a decreasing prostate-specific antigen (PSA) level. However, the patient also experienced substantial side effects that could have led to the end of treatment. We used our proprietary artificial intelligence (AI) technology, called CURATE.AI, to use only this patient's drug and dosing information to construct an individualized profile from which an optimal dose could be recommend to the clinical team, which represented an N-of-1 strategy for patient intervention. Following clinician approval, the drug doses were adjusted accordingly. Notably, CURATE.AI subsequently suggested a 50% reduction in drug dosage, which immediately led to the lowest recorded levels of PSA for this patient with tumor regression after 16 months.[23] Furthermore, the patient's subsequent dosing data were used to continuously update the profile, which resulted in dynamically adjusted dosing within established limits, representing a very different approach compared to traditional high- and fixed-dose therapy. As such, the treatment with the experimental drug combination combined with CURATE.AI dose optimization sustained treatment response and drug tolerability, ultimately improving the patient's quality of life as a result of lower side effects.

This case demonstrates the potential of personalizing medicine to achieve better health outcomes, and the applicability of this field stretches well beyond cancer. Chronic diseases, respiratory diseases, and multiple sclerosis, to name a few, could benefit from a more personalized approach as well.[24]

While N-of-1 strategies offer hope to patients in terms of individualizing care, the issues of scalability and financial sustainability are often at the forefront of discussions concerning the deployment potential of personalized medicine. When these issues are addressed by the technology itself and its pathway toward implementation, markedly reducing health care costs while providing equivalent or better health outcomes can potentially be achieved simultaneously.[25] Also, from an infrastructure requirement standpoint, this case study used a small data approach to individualize treatment that did not require large-scale population-wide data to inform the dosing process. With regard to outcomes, the risks of hospital admission for adverse events may have also been reduced. While further large-scale clinical and health care economics studies are underway or imminent, these and other considerations demonstrate the potential of harnessing scalable personalized medicine platforms as a means to improving the cost of care and treatment outcomes.

In summary, if DTx can provide better clinical and financial outcomes by taking a more personalized approach to many treatment pathways, the solution's economic impact is often a complex question that DTx innovators should not overlook. They will be required to demonstrate both the cost and the effectiveness of their solutions.

The Opportunity for DTx

Algorithms similar to CURATE.AI form an essential part of the engine that powers DTx. They incorporate hundreds of individual patient-level variables that provide visibility and insight into what a fully customized therapy for that particular patient may look like. You may recall our discussion in chapter 1 of the BlueStar® Insulin Adjustment Program, which enables diabetes patients to benefit from automated real-time adjustments to their insulin—that is a prime example of the power of DTx to improve patients' lives by taking the guesswork out of medication dosing. The ability of these strategies to empower patient adherence, which can in turn impact treatment outcomes and subsequent health system costs, cannot be overstated.

By harnessing DTx to realize N-of-1 interventions, it is possible to individualize and optimize care at the single-patient level, using their own data. This idea and its operationalization represent a game-changing shift in the way we approach health care and can lead to a genuinely personalized and scalable medicine, for better health outcomes and potentially lower costs.

DTx platforms have the potential to accelerate personalization in health care with customized algorithms, but also with more personalized interventions including behavioral change interventions. As we will see later, and continuing with diabetes as an example, patients using a DTx may be prompted to check their blood glucose in the mornings if the system realizes they have not been checking it regularly. They may also receive continuous real-time feedback, based on longer-term data patterns, of their own disease monitoring coupled with external information synthesized from a wide range of sources. Therefore, serial engagement with DTx could change the way we think about data in health care. For example, DTx-driven acquisition of longitudinal data could catalyze major advances in the types of data gleaned, the ease with which data are obtained, and how those data are acquired from individual patients. This collective shift in data acquisition is what will allow for DTx-centric, practice-changing advances in health care delivery.

Conclusion

The five questions outlined in this chapter are intended to guide DTx innovators and entrepreneurs in defining and prioritizing deficiencies in the current delivery and practice of health care, with an eye toward identifying which of these gaps digitization and technology are uniquely equipped to address. In this process, identifying the therapeutic areas with greatest unmet need and understanding the potential future consequences of not addressing those gaps, or not addressing them early enough, is of critical importance. Resolving some of them may require a prescription drug, medical device, or digital intervention, while others may not. Figuring out these intricacies and nuances may suggest different paths to commercialization with different partnerships and distribution models (i.e., with or without a pharmaceutical partnership). It will also influence the process of choosing a theoretical framework to guide the design and implementation of the DTx.

From our experience, this latter part of the process tends to be underestimated, despite the fact that a theoretical framework presents numerous benefits for the development, evaluation, and implementation of DTx.[26] For this reason, we asked Dr. Geck Hong Yeo, a scientist trained in the application of human development and psychological theories, and Matt Oon, CEO and founder of mental digital health company Acceset, to share their respective academic and entrepreneurial perspectives on how digital platforms can serve as a bridge between evidence-based theoretical frameworks and the design of therapeutic solutions (please see appendix B).

NOTES

1. Academy of Neurologic Music Therapy, "Academy Affiliate Roster by Name and Residence," accessed November 17, 2022, https://nmtacademy.co/findannmt. The Academy for Neurologic Music Therapy is an organization whose mission is to disseminate, advance, and protect the practice of neurologic music therapy worldwide.

2. Rossignol and Jones, "Audio-Spinal Influence in Man Studied by the H-Reflex and Its Possible Role on Rhythmic Movements Synchronized to Sound"; Trimble and Hesdorffer, "Music and the Brain: The Neuroscience of Music and Musical Appreciation."

3. Verghese et al., "Quantitative Gait Markers and Incident Fall Risk in Older Adults."

4. From an interview with the authors, December 8, 2020.

5. Van Oostrom et al., "Multimorbidity of Chronic Diseases and Health Care Utilization in General Practice."

6. World Health Organization, *Global Strategic Directions for Strengthening Nursing and Midwifery 2016–2020*.

7. Organisation for Economic Co-operation and Development, *Health at a Glance 2011: OECD Indicators*.

8. Resnikoff et al., "Estimated Number of Ophthalmologists Worldwide (International Council of Ophthalmology Update): Will We Meet the Needs?"

9. National Center for Advancing Translational Sciences, "About NCATS."

10. National Human Genome Research Institute, "Rare Diseases FAQ."

11. Angelis, Tordrup, and Kanavos, "Socio-Economic Burden of Rare Diseases."

12. Fraunhofer Institute for Algorithms and Scientific Computing SCAI, "Preventive Treatment for Alzheimer's and Parkinson's Disease"; Belluck and Robbins, "FDA Approves Alzheimer's Drug Despite Fierce Debate Over Whether It Works."

13. World Health Organization, "The Top 10 Causes of Death." Other diseases in this ranking include coronary artery disease; stroke; lower respiratory infections; chronic obstructive pulmonary disease; trachea, bronchus, and lung cancers; diabetes; dehydration due to diarrheal diseases; tuberculosis; and cirrhosis.

14. States, Pappas, and Salem, "Overground Physical Therapy Gait Training for Chronic Stroke Patients with Mobility Deficits."

15. Grefkes and Fink, "Recovery from Stroke: Current Concepts and Future Perspectives."

16. Choi et al., "Digital Therapeutics: Emerging New Therapy for Neurologic Deficits after Stroke."

17. David, Cristea, and Hofmann, "Why Cognitive Behavioral Therapy Is the Current Gold Standard of Psychotherapy."

18. American Psychological Association, "What Is Cognitive Behavioral Therapy?"

19. Kerr, "When Omada Health Was Young: The Early Years."

20. Adler and Page, Cancer Care for the Whole Patient; Naser et al., "Depression and Anxiety in Patients with Cancer"; Alagizy et al., "Anxiety, Depression, and Perceived Stress among Breast Cancer Patients."

21. Blue Note Therapeutics, "Cancer-Related Distress."

22. Luo et al., "A Comparison of Electronically Delivered and Face-to-Face Cognitive Behavioural Therapies in Depressive Disorders"; Fitzsimmons-Craft et al., "Effectiveness of a Digital Cognitive Behavior Therapy–Guided Self-Help Intervention for Eating Disorders in College Women."

23. Pantuck et al., "Modulating BET Bromodomain Inhibitor ZEN-3694 and Enzalutamide Combination Dosing in a Metastatic Prostate Cancer Patient using CURATE.AI, an Artificial Intelligence Platform."

24. Hult, Measuring the Potential Health Impact of Personalized Medicine; Noell, Faner, and Agustí, "From Systems Biology to P4 Medicine."

25. Kasztura et al., "Cost-Effectiveness of Precision Medicine."

26. Moller et al., "Applying and Advancing Behavior Change Theories and Techniques in the Context of a Digital Health Revolution"; Murray et al., "Evaluating Digital Health Interventions: Key Questions and Approaches"; Manta, Patrick-Lake, and Goldsack, "Digital Measures that Matter to Patients."

CHAPTER 4

Ensuring Business Viability Early

Please note that the "Financing Your Venture" section of this chapter was written with contributions by Benjamin Belot, partner at Kurma Partners, a European-based venture capitalist specializing in health care, including having two funds focused on therapeutics as well as on diagnosis and digital health.

As you further your understanding and exploration of important aspects of DTx development, sooner or later you are bound to have to tackle the question of business viability. Fully researching the conditions for the potential concept or venture's economic viability is particularly important for innovators and entrepreneurs who are trying to translate passion into a solid business proposition.

Ensuring the business viability of any new venture—not just DTx—always starts by mapping out the growth projections and defining what needs to be true for the business model to reach the desired milestones and targets. Concepts such as the total addressable market (TAM), serviceable available market (SAM), and serviceable obtainable market (SOM) are considered the fundamental market size metrics and are a good starting point.[1] Studying these concepts and backing them with market research will validate the market potential for your concept. Is there a potential market and could it be served in a way that turns your innovation into a profitable business (e.g., economic viability)? Is it worth your time and resources? Could it be an investment opportunity for potential investors?

Investors will want to see that you have done your research and set ambitious but *realistic* revenue goals (and not the biggest possible numbers). In addition to the TAM, SAM, and SOM, there are many tools and frameworks out there that can help you in assessing whether there is a real revenue opportunity available for your venture. We are not going to list them all. Instead, in this chapter we introduce one of the simplest yet most powerful tools to use early in your journey: the reverse income statement (figure 4.1).

The reverse income statement should affirm that you are moving in the right direction and confirm the business viability of addressing the problem with the tool you identified per the previous chapters. The premise of the reverse income statement is to "envision the unknown" via "discovery-driven planning" applied to strategy, business, and marketing of a new venture.[2] It starts by determining the target profit margin or annual profits for your venture (first cell on the left); this is typically a measure of profitability over three years or five years. This first assumption depends on your solution and an initial business plan that reflects your TAM, SAM, and SOM.

In an example of hypothetical company Newco Inc., focusing on stroke survivors and chronic pain management in the United States, we have set an annual profit goal of $5 million by year five, which is a rather ambitious profitability target considering that most digital ventures focus on customer acquisition and top-line growth to drive a company's sales and revenues. As a result, you may want to start using the reverse income statement by determining your target annual revenues first. Otherwise, after defining the profitability target, simply work backward to define annual revenues and operating costs. For Newco Inc., we assumed a 50% gross profit margin. (For reference, target gross profit margins hover around 80% for digital health

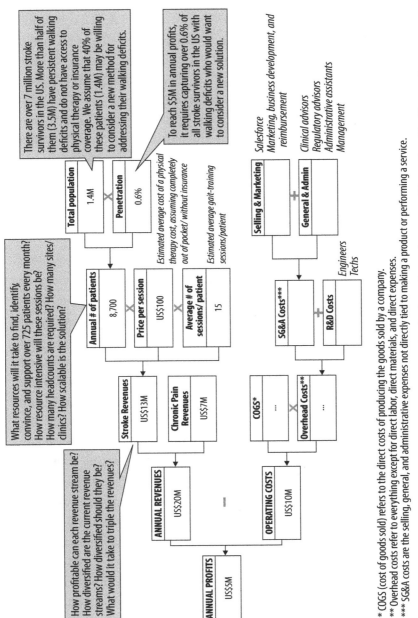

FIGURE 4.1. An example of a reverse income statement for the hypothetical company Newco Inc. (for illustration purposes only). What needs to come true for Newco to reach $5 million in annual profits by year five? Source: From the authors

* COGS (cost of goods sold) refers to the direct costs of producing the goods sold by a company.
** Overhead costs refer to everything except for direct labor, direct materials, and direct expenses.
*** SG&A costs are the selling, general, and administrative expenses not directly tied to making a product or performing a service.

company Livongo[3] and 60% for both telehealth company Teladoc[4] and medtech company Medtronic.[5]) Continue to work backward on the reverse income statement and assume Newco Inc. has two main service lines coming from stroke survivors with walking deficits (revenue stream #1) and from persons with chronic pain (revenue stream #2). At some point we arrive at the near future, where we can compare the inferred state of your business with what is realistically achievable.

The reverse income statement forces you to make assumptions, define what success would look like, and therefore define the basic economics of the business. Essentially you need to ask yourself, "What needs to happen to achieve the outcomes I am (or my investor is) seeking?" It could be a series of interim goals in terms of the number of users, the number of providers, the potential uptake of a new solution, or other factors for your venture to be viable. Finally, link these desired outcomes to what might drive them.

The more assumptions you make, the more complex your reverse income statement will be. Stress test each assumption with a what-if scenario in order to visualize how situations outside your control—such as economic changes to the health care system, new health care regulations, or current events (e.g., global pandemics)—might impact your plan. We also recommend attaching corresponding activities and milestones that you would need to reach for those assumptions to come true. For example, if you are concerned about your ability to reach a certain number of clinics that serve a certain number of patients in a given year, it may help to define what would it take to secure a single clinic in terms of resources (e.g., manpower and marketing efforts required), success ratio (i.e., for one clinic you may need to engage 10 other clinics), lead time (i.e., how long would it take you to convert a single clinic from a prospect to a customer, gaining their willingness to prescribe your solution), and so on. In short, have a detailed plan.

Working through the hypothetical example in figure 4.1, one would conclude that reaching the target gross profit margin of $5 million by year five would require serving over 700 stroke survivors with walking deficits every month, in addition to the pain management patients we didn't factor in for this example. Is this logistically feasible? Technically possible? Based on this analysis, reaching the target profit level requires serving the vast majority of Newco's total population (i.e., its total addressable market). These are the patients who could potentially benefit from the solution in a given market, country, or city within a limited period (and probably limited financial resources). Therefore, Newco's concept and go-to-market plan are unlikely to be feasible.

Keep in mind that there are other planning tools besides the reverse income statement one can use to assess the business viability of a DTx concept. If you are interested in learning more about them, we recommend you take a look at the following:

- *Pro forma operations specs*, which lay out the operations needed to produce, sell, service, and deliver a service to an end user— in other words, the activities required to run the business;
- *Key assumptions checklist*, which aids to ensure that assumptions are checked and validated; and
- *Milestone planning chart*, which specifies the assumptions to be tested at each project milestone.[6]

Our focus in the Newco example was on driving profitability, but we understand that the success of your venture and potential investors may not be solely defined by profitability. It's important to consider the competitive dynamics of your industry. In a new area like DTx, where market education is required, there may be a need to buy into the market and establish dominance at the expense of short run profitability in order to become the market leader. Keep this in mind as you use some of the tools mentioned in this chapter.

Financing Your Venture

At this stage of your DTx development, you probably have a good idea of how big your company should be within the next two to three years (e.g., number of employees, number of products, etc.), as well as your patient and physician acquisition strategy and costs. Soon after determining the market potential and business viability of your solution, you will need to start thinking about raising capital to support your budding company. In the startup world, this usually entails organizing your first round of funding, onboarding investors, and developing the capacity to think not only as a CEO with a growth mindset, but also as a CFO looking at the financial management of the venture. Since we are talking about startups and we have covered a diverse range of topics that drive innovation, you may also need to be prepared to think simultaneously from many other perspectives, ranging from operations to business development and beyond.

How to Choose the Right Investor for Your Startup

Regardless of your venture's development stage, getting investors on board is an important decision for any entrepreneur. It goes beyond the financial aspects, often addressing the entrepreneur's concerns about the potential dilution of control too early.[7] You may have heard this before, but it's worth saying again: ideal investors should represent a lot more than a check. Funding your startup should be focused on how investors will add value to you and your team, as well as how their investment would accelerate and derisk your growth plan. We invite you to consider the following two questions when choosing the investors:

What assets, capabilities, and resources would the investors bring in? The investors' networks and their ability to facilitate introductions are often the most tangible short-term benefits to a startup. Entrepreneurs should also look for complementary expertise that investors with experience in health care, technology, or business can bring to the table. This relates to our previous mention that DTx should be the best of these three worlds. So what expertise is the most critical to your venture in order to advance to the next round of funding? Does this critical expertise include clinical trial design and initiation, obtaining regulatory approvals and reimbursement, or perhaps how to form a partnership with a larger pharmaceutical company? What expertise do you already have in your team and what are you missing?

How well would you work with the investors? The relationship between a startup founder and investors can be complex, but keep in mind that both of you have the same goal at the end of the day: to see your venture grow and make an impact, both clinically and financially. The paths to get there may be different as your ambitions and appetite for risk may differ. Expectations and values must be aligned early on to get the right chemistry. Investors should be considered as partners because they share your vision and also because some are likely to join your company's board of directors. Choosing the right investor is akin to choosing the next member of your leadership team.

Similar to how you have a few rounds of discussions before selecting members of your C-suite, it is important to do your research and due diligence on these potential partner investors as well. What kind of companies have they supported in the past? How did they support them and how could they support you? What kind of expectations would they have—from the more strategic considerations, such as being on your board, potential veto rights, and so on, to the more tactical aspects, such as what kind of reporting are they expecting? Different investors have different collaboration models. Some will want to be involved in the day-to-day operations while others prefer to be more hands-off and wait for a return on investment. Discussions with them should focus on how they can assist you in validating, executing, and accelerating your growth strategy, and also on what type of decision power they expect during the course of operations, rather than how deep their pockets are. In short, be clear about your needs and what type of partnership you want with your investors.

What to Know Before Talking to an Investor

Have a robust roadmap. At this stage of your venture development, your plan should include, for example, your paths to generate regulatory-grade clinical evidence. Kaia Health, a DTx that focuses on musculo-skeletal disorders, is a good example of generating early evidence as the funding came in. The company was launched in 2016 with US$4 million in seed funding. In 2017 and 2018, they published two obser-vational studies.[8] A year later, they successfully raised US$18 million in series A and published outcomes from their first randomized con-trolled trial (RCT) of 101 patients.[9] In 2020, they raised another US$26 million and published their second RCT results with 1,245 patients.[10] As in the case of Kaia, generating robust clinical evidence is critical to achieving a scalable business model and the success of you and your investor. For an example of how a digital health solution can be grounded in evidence-based theories and techniques, see appendix B. Evidence-based DTx platforms tend to be more effective than those that are not, and in short, they can make the difference between a me-ticulously designed DTx "star" and a hastily put together DTx "flop."

Stand out from the crowd. As we defined in the first chapter, a DTx is not a simple mobile app or a digital version of established therapy pro-grams. Those could be a starting point, but not the end point. The importance of demonstrating efficacy through human trials (i.e., RCTs) goes hand-in-hand with the importance of developing proprietary solutions. Your startup's intellectual property (IP) portfolio plays a cru-cial role in protecting its competitive advantage, in differentiating from existing or alternative solutions, and in supporting future invest-ments. As Brian Harris, cofounder and CEO of MedRhythms men-tioned, "Building a strong IP portfolio is an integral part of our strategy to build a large, defensible and successful company that makes a big impact in the world."[11]

If DTx can be protected in a manner similar to that of traditional therapeutics, these competitive edges should not be limited to patentable opportunities. A state-of-the-art interface for a unique, engaging, and sustainable user experience, dedicated solutions to caregivers and physicians, or a unique business model based on a portfolio approach of complementary DTx solutions can also create unique competitive advantages for DTx organizations.

In short, as you define your growth plan you will need to have an investment strategy to raise capital. Doing your research to determine what kind of investor your company needs and how they can contribute to the growth of your venture is critical. The founder-investor relationship is not solely based on money. For investors, the return on investment is considered an "output" as a result of the relationship (or investment) with you. They would most likely want to have a say in the "inputs" and track nonfinancial metrics related to the clinical validation, clinical buy-in, customer acquisition, engagement, and their experience, as well as the DTx's overall traction in the market and revenue trajectory. Startup fundraising requires building relationships with investors, so be prepared to put in time and resources to achieve this critically important step.

NOTES

1. Total addressable market (also called total available market) refers to the total revenue opportunity available for a product or service. Serviceable available market is the total market demand for a product or service, the part of the total addressable market that can actually be reached. Serviceable obtainable market, also referred to as the share of market, is the estimated portion of revenue within a specific product segment that you are able capture.

2. McGrath and MacMillan, "Discovery-Driven Planning."

3. Livongo Health, "Livongo Reports Third Quarter 2020 Financial Results."

4. Teladoc Health, "Teladoc Health Reports Third-Quarter 2020 Results."

5. "Medtronic Profit Margin 2006–2021," *Macrotrends*.

6. McGrath and MacMillan, "Discovery-Driven Planning."

7. Dilution of control refers to the decrease in existing shareholder-ownership percentages of a company, also known as equity dilution, which often translates to

a potential lack of control as the founder, entrepreneur, or CEO over your company's future. It's a concern for entrepreneurs but also a potential red flag for early investors.

8. Huber et al., "Treatment of Low Back Pain with a Digital Multidisciplinary Pain Treatment App"; Clement et al., "Implementing Systematically Collected User Feedback to Increase User Retention in a Mobile App for Self-Management of Low Back Pain."

9. Toelle et al., "App-Based Multidisciplinary Back Pain Treatment versus Combined Physiotherapy Plus Online Education."

10. Priebe et al., "Digital Treatment of Back Pain versus Standard of Care."

11. MedRhythms, "MedRhythms Announces an Expansion of Intellectual Property Portfolio, Securing Patent on Audio Engine for Digital Therapeutics Platform."

CHAPTER 5

Test, Learn, and Pivot

At this stage, you may have more questions than answers, more suppositions than confirmations, about potential therapeutic areas of focus, the profile of your would-be customers and their motivations, the price to put on your DTx, and the exact structure of your DTx business model. For this reason, it is important as a DTx innovator and entrepreneur to embrace a culture of "test and learn" from day one. Commit to refining your envisioned solution and its potential application as you gain new insights and user[1] feedback.

While you may already have a plan to test, validate, and optimize the assumptions you have made during the discovery stage, there are more steps needed to achieve success in this space. Leading a DTx venture includes being prepared to face the unknowns (i.e., address gaps or blind spots in your assumptions that you may not have expected) and to pivot strategically when required. As business author Leon C. Megginson says, "It is not the most intellectual of the species that survives; it is not the strongest that survives, but the species that survives is the one that is able best to adapt and adjust to the changing environment in which it finds itself."[2] In other words, the species that survive are those that are most flexible and responsive to change. If we regard DTx organizations as a "species" of health care organizations, figuratively speaking, we could say that those who adopt a test-and-learn culture stand the greatest chance of developing great products. This culture entails having processes in place that empower teams to continuously and dynamically optimize their products based on new learnings.

Take for example, Google.com, which exists in many people's minds as a source for all answers. The truth is, even within the company itself, employees are always searching, testing, and learning how to deliver better search outcomes. In one instance, Google was notably unable to decide between which shades of blue to use for advertising links in Gmail and Google Search. This led to a test called, with tongue in cheek, "Fifty Shades of Blue." The technology giant showed 41 different shades of blue to approximately 2% of its users and found that a slightly purple shade of blue maximized the likelihood of users clicking on the links. Unexpectedly, the slight change in color generated an extra US$200 million a year in advertisement revenue for the company. How's that for continuous learning?

Humana Inc., an American health care insurance provider, is another example demonstrating the importance of testing, learning, and pivoting. Humana wanted to optimize the first thing visitors see when visiting their homepage—the main banner. Such banners are important as they create a focus point that captures the interest of visitors with an objective to encourage them to stay on the website for further browsing, or to click on it to learn about the displayed product and ultimately generate purchase orders. In business jargon, we call it "lead generation." Humana ran two tests, comparing a "control" banner and an optimized "treatment" banner, with different messages, pictures, and so on, to see which banner had a greater ability to generate click-throughs. The treatment banners resulted in 433% more and 192% more clicks for the first and second tests, respectively, reflecting a better ability than the control banners to catch more of the visitors' attention and curiosity in Humana's solutions.

The type of testing both Google and Humana undertook is known as A/B testing—a process of controlled experimentation whereby different variations of a product or service are served randomly to users to determine the highest-performing variation.[3] If it worked for Google and Humana, it can also work for DTx organizations.

What Should We Test?

If your background in product development is in a field unrelated to health care or DTx, you can still apply your know-how to this new innovation terrain. In this case, you should strive to avoid the so-called curse of knowledge, a cognitive bias when we fail to properly understand the perspective of those who do not have as much information as we do and may require a learning process in order to sufficiently contribute toward innovation and the productization processes. Deep-rooted assumptions based on past experience working in another sector or with a narrow group of constituents do not necessarily translate into an intuitive understanding of the unique job to be done or how to address the jobs of the various stakeholders along the DTx value chain.

If you have no background or prior experience in product development, and this DTx project is your first entrepreneurship endeavor, you would want to accelerate your learning curve in order to get up to speed faster and realize the full potential of your DTx solution.

Regardless of where you stand between these extremes on the innovation spectrum—whether you are a veteran or a newcomer—derisking your strategy and business model by testing key assumptions early will be essential.[4] Examples of typical assumptions you may wish to test include:

- Would physicians be willing to prescribe my DTx?
- Would patients be willing to pay x amount of money for a digitally delivered therapeutic?
- How comfortable would users be with a particular feature?
- What role would caregivers play in the care continuum?
- Would payers be willing to implement new risk-sharing models?

To test your assumptions in an organized way, we suggest sorting them across three categories—*test now*, *test next*, and *test later*—depending on how critical you believe the findings to be for your strategy and business model.

To illustrate the test-and-learn approach to developing a DTx solution, let us consider the experience of AEvice Health, a Singapore-based medtech company addressing chronic respiratory diseases. AEvice's offering is a smart, wearable patch attached to a child's chest that acts as a digital stethoscope to track the child's respiratory and heart rates during sleep, which is particularly relevant for managing asthma. Within three months of starting the company, and with seed investment under US$5,000, the team launched multiple A/B testing campaigns on social media to help it figure out and fine-tune the following domains:

- *Strategic focus areas*: potential "verticals," or use cases. These include the applications of the technology to address different conditions, including asthma.
- *Value proposition*: optimal strategies to articulate the product's potential benefits to different profiles of intended users. For example, the team explored different taglines, such as "able to care," "recording your symptoms," and "peace of mind."
- *Pricing*: finding and testing the sweet spot between a would-be customer's willingness to pay for the solution and the investment the company would need to conduct online user research and marketing in order to identify and convince potential buyers.
- *Call to action*: using different marketing campaigns and messaging to encourage website visitors to take the desired action, such as "subscribe today" or "download now." In addition, AEvice tested their website visitors' willingness to leave their email address to receive future updates. This action was an important part of the test as one may like an advertisement but may not necessarily be interested in buying the product. A customer leaving their email address is therefore one more data point toward gauging user interest.

The AEvice team obtained thousands of data points from the potential users through the online A/B testing. It also interviewed some of the individuals who had provided their email addresses. As Adrian Ang, the cofounder of AEvice said, "None of us are marketing trained. It was our first step toward doing market research. These experiments helped us refine our targeted customer profiles[7] and their motivations, and also confirmed some of our business model's assumptions." In short, the research helped the company to understand the needs and expectations of its potential customers to derisk the journey ahead.

Understanding how much potential customers are willing to spend on your solution (a concept known as "willingness to pay"), independently of your future go-to-market approaches and commercialization strategies (see chapters 11 and 12), merits evaluation. To address this point, AEvice turned to social media engagement, which then strengthened its business case when engaging with potential strategic and channel partners later in its product journey.

Case Study: A Personal Experience Testing Digital Health Potential for Early Dementia Screening in Japan

A few years ago, while working with a leading insurance company client in Japan, a member of our WisDM team was tasked with exploring the potential launch of a digital health solution for early dementia screening. A traditional route would have been to conduct lengthy market research that would have cost the client anywhere between US$50K and US$100K. Instead, with the insurer's health innovation team, a test-and-learn approach was used to test the assumptions and local utility of the concept, which would be much less expensive while yielding more robust insights compared to the traditional route.

The process started off by examining the typical experience of patients living with dementia, as well as the experiences of other such relevant stakeholders as physicians and insurance agents. In interviews with patients, there was a particular interest in pinpointing the specific moment when they first recognized the symptoms of dementia and when they got diagnosed, as well as understanding the emotions associated with those moments. Commonalities across the interviewed patient journeys to identify recurring pain points were also explored. Armed with those insights, the team generated over 30 assumptions about patient desire to understand and assess their dementia risk level, as well as their willingness to take action to prevent or delay the onset of dementia. Ideating and testing these assumptions then formed the basis of a potential scalable digital health solution that spots early signs of dementia.

Test 1: Gauging Interest

The first test launched a Facebook campaign that showed randomly selected users an invitation to participate in a dementia-related quiz. Similar to Humana's approach to optimize their website banner, different messages and images for this campaign were used to continuously collect such data as click-through rates (CTRs), cost-per-click, quiz completion, and cost-per-completion.

Within five days on a modest budget, the team collected more than 300 high dimensional data points. Additional analysis led the team to conclude that Facebook users in Japan had a strong interest in knowing more about dementia, as suggested by a fivefold-higher CTR for the messages from the study as compared to the industry benchmark. The team also concluded that positively framed messages had higher CTR than negatively framed ones and that potentially threatening terms such as *worried*, *concerned*, and *confused* should be avoided in future marketing materials. Additionally, rather than the term *dementia*, *brain health* emerged as the preferred concept as it was easier to spark a discussion around this topic, particularly with healthy or nondiagnosed individuals.

Through hundreds of quiz responses, the team concluded that in general there was a lack of understanding and knowledge about dementia. Respondents in Japan also showed a strong interest in assessing their cognitive risk as early as possible and were more receptive of words such as *preventive* rather than *reactive*. Respondents were also seeking guidance on cognitive risk assessment, such as how to detect potential early signs of dementia and when it was advisable to see a doctor, rather than waiting for a dementia diagnosis when preemptive action was possible.

Lastly, the team collected valuable insights on the demographic profiles and personas of potential customers who seemed most receptive to messaging around dementia-related solutions. This helped the team obtain a deeper understanding of the optimal population segment to which a dementia DTx could be targeted. Thus, test 1 revealed the most relevant assumptions about would-be customers' concerns around dementia, while also confirming that there was a need in the market for a dementia diagnostic solution.

Test 2: Monetization Paths

In a second test, the team wanted to explore ways in which an insurance company could monetize this potential new DTx offering. At the time, most DTx solutions that fell under the category of value-added services were complementary to core insurance products, and the team's goal was to evaluate whether the added value of a DTx solution would make prospective customers more likely to buy the core product.

The team tested this concept by promoting a DTx solution on social media to see whether it could generate leads on who would buy an insurance product if it came paired with a DTx. The team created what is known in product management as a "painted door test"—an approach that lets developers gauge interest in a product or service before it's built. They put together a landing page on the topic of brain health to validate whether a user would be interested enough in learning more about the DTx to submit their contact information. If they did, this opened the door to building further relationships with those users as prospective customers.

Within a few days of the painted door test, the team realized that the CTR on the landing page was over 10 times higher than the industry standard. Inversely, the investment required to collect contact information per prospective customer was 20-60 times lower than the insurance industry average at the time in Japan, confirming that social media and the deployed mechanisms were a promising avenue for lead acquisition.

The two experiments pertaining to introducing a dementia screening digital health solution on the Japanese market demonstrated not only how creative and agile DTx organizations can be in terms of generating and testing their assumptions, but also how social media, where appropriate, can be leveraged to do so.

Beyond A/B Testing

Attrition rate (the number of people who initiate an intervention and later abandon it) is a critical variable for an effective intervention that requires a sustained user engagement. According to a systematic review of 22 randomized clinical trials, assessing the impact of digital health interventions on health-related outcomes in the workplace, the attrition rates were as high as 60%, with a median rate of 21%, suggesting that sustaining engagement is a challenge for digital health solutions.[8] This realization should lead DTx innovators to ask themselves five key questions:

- *About utility*: Does the therapeutic address the unmet needs and jobs to be done of physicians and patients?
- *About usability*: Are customers able to use the solution easily?
- *About sustainability*: Will customers adhere to use by returning to the solution?
- *About desirability*: Do customers like the way the solution looks and feels?
- *About branding*: What are the customers' overall feelings about the solution and brand?

These questions can be tested in different ways. Below we list four types of strategic experiments you can consider, which are from *The Innovator's Guide to Growth*[9] and were utilized in collaboration with Innosight, a management consulting company:

- *Concept tests* are used to pitch solutions to different groups of stakeholders, using verbal descriptions as well as audiovisual materials, such as sketches, models, and video clips of the hypothesized user experience. The audiovisual elements help stakeholders visualize the potential concept and bring the idea to life, enabling them to give more accurate feedback on which solutions are likely to work and how they can be improved. A concept test could also show mock-ups of a DTx interface to gather qualitative insights from potential users.
- *Functioning prototypes* are tangible and experiential models of the envisioned solution. By observing how stakeholders interact with them, and assessing features that may drive sustained interaction, developers can gain a better understanding of how well the proposed solution and key features deliver against the jobs to be done. Feedback and learning can be captured through iterative stakeholder interactions as the prototypes get increasingly refined.
- In *transaction tests*, the offering is presented to customers for consideration and purchase in a setting that mimics the natural purchase environment. There is no better way to substantiate the viability of a new business model than recreating real-world transactions to determine if customers would pay for the solution.
- *Operational pilots* are used to provide real in-market learning within a scaled-down environment. It allows the team to validate some of the most important assumptions around marketing, distribution, repeated purchases, and resource requirements, which are hard to test until the solution is made available to a big enough market for a long enough period of time.

Go Further with Multivariate and Factorial Testing

A range of test designs can shed important insight on the mechanisms driving user interactions with DTx. Compared to A/B tests, multivariate tests compare a higher number of variables, revealing insights that can only be gleaned from understanding how these variables interact with one another. In addition, factorial experiments can infer interaction spaces between the tested factors by assessing a small number of carefully selected combinations. For example, a factorial design experiment was used to identify effective intervention components for a smoking cessation program. The study tested six intervention components: nicotine patch vs. no intervention (none); nicotine gum vs. none; counseling vs. none; intensive cessation in-person counseling vs. minimal; intensive cessation phone counseling vs. minimal; and 16 vs. 8 weeks of combination nicotine replacement therapy.[10] Through this test, performed with carefully selected combinations of factors, the researchers concluded that preparation counseling and the combination of intensive cessation in-person counseling with preparation nicotine gum or patch were promising intervention components for smoking and should be evaluated as an integrated treatment package.

As the examples from Google, AEvice, and the dementia case study in Japan show, for any of the tests mentioned here, and for product development overall, a recommended practice is to develop and test the assumptions with the would-be end users. Designing a product that is wanted by its user base can then be built using the test-and-learn approach and the following best practices:[11]

- Design the product using a human-centered approach, accounting for the user's core needs, abilities, and environments of use, and device interface.
- Design the product to optimize adoption, engagement, and adherence within the target population.
- Integrate product accessibility and universally designed features where appropriate.

- Conduct human factors testing throughout the product development and usability processes.

From ideation to commercialization and post-marketing software upgrades, the most impactful and enduring DTx solutions will be those that undergo constant improvement based on input from the larger deployment ecosystem. This ecosystem, as well as its criteria for adherence, can be dynamic, changing over time both across users and even for the same user. Hence, a test-and-learn culture throughout the organization should be part of any ambitious DTx company's DNA, as proven by the most advanced technology firms. For this feedback loop to work, DTx innovators must therefore build mechanisms that enable frequent testing and evaluation into the development cycle of their product and maintain these processes from prototyping all the way through to post-market release phases.

Conclusion

When piloting DTx solutions in day-to-day care, it is critical to continuously test and validate the solution itself and its business model with evolving use contexts. The tools, behavioral models, and techniques presented in this chapter should be a starting point to help your organization overcome some of the most common challenges faced by DTx organizations at this stage and get you on track to move from pilot to production.

NOTES
1. We prefer the term *user*, or *end user*, over *patient* to refer to the person who is ultimately going to use the DTx as it could be patients themselves or caregivers, physicians, or any health care professionals.
2. Megginson, "Lessons from Europe for American Business."
3. Young, "Improving Library User Experience with A/B Testing."
4. There are risks inherent in launching any venture. They can be risks related to the product, your business model, the team you are going to hire, investors you are to let join the board, and so on. Being involved in a DTx venture will come with specific risks and uncertainties related to the nature of the technology evolving in

a complex environment. New pathways need to be created (e.g., regulatory and reimbursement approvals) and many questions have not being completely addressed yet (e.g., physicians or patients buy-in for such new solutions). Therefore, an important part in being successful in developing, validating, and implementing a DTx is about managing these risks, trying to define, analyze, and anticipate them. In short, it's about derisking your venture's strategy and overall business model. As we use this term, *derisking*, throughout the book, we will suggest how others have done it and suggest recommendations.

5. World Health Organization, "Asthma: Key Facts."

6. World Health Organization, "Asthma: Key Facts."

7. This is independently if you are going the business-to-business (BTB) route, where a health care practitioner will prescribe the DTx solution to a patient or a business organization will make your solution available to the end user (e.g., employers for their employees), or the business-to-consumers (BTC) route, where you are serving directly the end user of the solution, through an online e-commerce platform, for example.

8. Howarth et al., "The Impact of Digital Health Interventions on Health-Related Outcomes in the Workplace."

9. Anthony et al., *The Innovator's Guide to Growth*.

10. Piper et al., "Identifying Effective Intervention Components for Smoking Cessation."

11. Digital Therapeutics Alliance, *DTx Product Best Practices*.

PART III

FROM PILOT TO PRODUCTION

Thinking beyond the Algorithm

Our ethos at WisDM states, "Technology alone cannot change health care." It is a particularly important consideration when the technology is transferred from proof of concept into standard of care. As Dr. Carolyn Lam pointed out in the introduction, "It's not because you have an algorithm that you have a commercial-ready product. We should not underestimate the amount of work that it takes to integrate with existing electronic medical records, fix data silos, design the right interface, protect patient data, and get all the regulatory approvals." During this part of the DTx journey, it is important for DTx entrepreneurs to have not only the "right" algorithm but also the "right" product that can be integrated successfully into everyday clinical practice.

In this section of the book, we walk you through the steps required to overcome common DTx implementation challenges, starting with the importance of addressing aspects of data sourcing and management (chapter 6). We also touch upon the critical importance of generating evidence and exploring novel approaches to clinical validation (chapter 7).

Variability in Care Delivery

Pilot studies aim to preliminarily examine specific variables of interest pertaining to a candidate intervention. These preliminary studies can determine if larger, sufficiently powered studies are warranted, or to potentially refine trial designs should the study be expanded. Pilot studies are usually conducted under controlled conditions, which can help to isolate and generate conclusions about these variables. However, results from pilot studies may not fully represent all the nuances and circumstances of delivering care to patients in a routine, real-life setting—often termed *real-world data*. It is important for DTx entrepreneurs to understand this limitation and why interventions with promising outcomes from pilots do not always translate into routine clinical practice.

"Many promising technological innovations in health and social care are characterized by non-adoption or abandonment by individuals, or by failed attempts to scale up locally, spread distantly, or sustain the innovation long term at the organization or system level," says Trish Greenhalgh, a British primary care practitioner, academic, and one of the world's foremost experts in research translation.[1] This challenge expands much deeper into the complexities of clinical practice beyond an introduction of a new technology. Even with the highest level of evidence backing the proposed solution, cementing change in clinical practice is not easy. Let's consider two distinct studies looking at adherence to national guidelines— that is, best clinical practice recommendations based on evidence and agreed on at a national level to lead to the most optimal results.[2]

In a study performed in the United States, Dr. Elizabeth A. McGlynn and her team of researchers telephoned a random sample of over 20,000 adults over a two-year period and asked them about their health care experiences. The researchers also reviewed the patients' medical records and evaluated the quality of care the patients had received using 439 indicators for 30 acute and chronic conditions (such as diabetes, hypertension, and cancer) as well as preventive interventions (such as mammography screening for breast cancer, screening for cervical cancer, or having smoking status documented). The study found that only 55% of patients received the type and level of medical care recommended by national guidelines[3] for their conditions, with substantial variability between conditions, ranging from 78.7% of recommended care for senile cataract to 10.5% for alcohol dependence.[4] In short, the study revealed a substantial gap in the care as recommended to be provided and as received by the individuals, suggesting suboptimal adherence to standard health care guidelines by the medical professionals.

Suboptimal adherence to standard health care treatment guidelines is not specific to the United States. Another recent study performed in Australia examined whether health care for children aged 15 years and younger was consistent with established quality standards. The study assessed the clinical records for 17 high-incidence child health conditions (such as asthma and type 1 diabetes) and estimated the overall adherence to be 59.8%, with substantial variation across conditions. Taking asthma as an example, guidelines for the management of asthma recommend that each child receive a *written* action plan. This recommendation was followed for approximately 47% of the children assessed by this study who were prescribed an asthma inhaler.[5]

Awareness of a variability in provider adherence to national guidelines and evidence-based practice overall is a starting point to understanding factors that influence the implementation of new technologies and why beyond pilots, full-scale adoption of technologies, including DTx remains a challenge.

Implementation Science

As we stated earlier, our innovation ethos is that technology alone cannot transform health care. Beyond the ideation and validation of promising technologies, there remains a critical need to develop a road map toward successful deployment of these ideas into clinical practice to catalyze broad adoption across providers through patient communities. After all, highly innovative, evidence-backed technologies that cause inconveniences to clinical workflows may end up not being adopted. This is where domains such as implementation science (IS), defined as the scientific study of methods to promote the systematic uptake of research findings and other evidence-based practices into routine practice, become essential. Many successful scale-up programs are based upon the principles of IS,[6] which provides a useful lens to understand key considerations for introducing DTx into new care delivery settings that should be top-of-mind for DTx entrepreneurs and innovators.

Based on our own experience, interviews with digital health and DTx CEOs, and the published evidence, implementing and sustaining DTx (or any technology) in health care is a complex undertaking. We therefore look at leveraging the factors that influence the successful implementation of new technologies in chapter 8. We will also offer a how-to approach to implementing DTx, following the IS approach and offer the perspective of health care system managers on DTx integration in chapter 9. Finally, we discuss how DTx entrepreneurs might use behavioral methods like "nudging" to gain clinical buy-in and patient acceptance in chapter 10.

Technology-driven innovation moves at an extraordinarily fast pace, much faster than a health care system's readiness to integrate this technology into existing infrastructures, processes, and cultural norms. This misalignment applies to DTx too. We believe that during the transition from a DTx prototype to pilot study, and ultimately to commercial product innovation and real-world data generation, the innovators should be guided by a structured approach to identify and address the substantial challenges of changing clinical practice at scale.

NOTES

1. Greenhalgh et al., "Beyond Adoption: A New Framework for Theorizing and Evaluating Nonadoption, Abandonment, and Challenges to the Scale-Up, Spread, and Sustainability of Health and Care Technologies."

2. Frequently used as a measure to determine the quality of care.

3. Guidelines are used for clinical decision-making and reduce practice variation to ultimately improve patient outcomes.

4. McGlynn et al., "The Quality of Health Care Delivered to Adults in the United States."

5. Braithwaite et al., "Quality of Health Care for Children in Australia, 2012–2013."

6. Greenhalgh and Papoutsi, "Spreading and Scaling up Innovation and Improvement."

CHAPTER 6

Data Sourcing and Management

Collecting and managing medical data is not a trivial task. It requires substantial infrastructure, capital, expertise, trust, and time. You will experience the complexity of working with medical data throughout your DTx journey. The first touchpoint—data sourcing—is when you source medical data to test and demonstrate the basis for your idea. The second touchpoint—data management—is when you have the data under your purview, either sourced externally or collected by your platform.

When you approach a dataset owner to negotiate access to the data, be prepared to discuss the extent of that access and who will own the data processing products (that is, your analytical tool and the data analysis results). Additionally, once you start analyzing the data, you are responsible for the data stewardship—ensuring the privacy of the individuals who contributed to the dataset and the security of their information. Once your platform starts collecting and generating the data itself, you need to ensure that appropriate measures are in place to do the same for the newly collected data.

Questions spanning not only technology but also ethics and legislation will certainly arise throughout your quest to secure access to the type of medical data on which your DTx will run and to identify the right framework and processing rules for managing those type of sourced and newly collected data. In this chapter, we provide you with a detailed overview of the most common medical data sources and outline key considerations around data ownership and stewardship.

DTx-Relevant Data and Where to Find Them

One of the most common types of data used for training and testing medical software is deidentified retrospective medical datasets, which contain patient medical history (diagnoses, visit notes, and treatment courses) with such patient identifiers as names and social security numbers removed. Aspiring DTx startups have several options to obtain access to these datasets:

1. Access theme-specific, publicly available data repositories (also known as *data commons*), which may or may not include accompanying analytical tools and are open for anyone to use in the spirit of open science. Those datasets are often the output of research projects that have been funded with the requirement to publish their data processing products and results.
2. Participate in private (e.g., corporate- or insurer-sponsored) and public (e.g., hospital- or university-organized) innovation events and incubator programs specifically aimed at startups that enable them to access data governed by these institutions. Of note: participating in such events may require physical attendance at the institutions' premises (e.g., institutional incubator programs).
3. Join data consortia that allow for data usage without interfering with ownership or governance (e.g., multiparty computation networks). This can usually be done remotely but will likely be subject to consortia-specific guidelines and contracting.
4. Buy access to medical data (e.g., for-profit datasets). In these cases, data sourcing and ownership should be carefully vetted to ensure their ethical sourcing, quality, and reliability.

As you can see, there are multiple sources where one can find medical data. However, while finding *a* data source may not seem too challenging, finding the *right* data source is a different story. What is the difference between the two and what it does it mean for you?

How to Identify a High-Quality Data Source

The right data source should provide data of high quality and relevance to the patient population your solution is designed for. This is because your data processing products (DPP)—which comprise the tool, software, and technology developed and refined with the data found in your chosen data source, and the end results of the data analysis performed with that tool—will ultimately serve as the evidence backing your idea, and they can be only as good as the quality of the data at their foundation. Therefore, if the data are of poor quality, so will your DPP. These considerations are echoed in our conversation with Dr. Kee Yuan Ngiam, Group Chief Technology Officer of the National University Health System in Singapore[1]—a key type of stakeholder with whom a DTx organization may engage toward the deployment of its platform at a large health care system: "Our collaboration with potential partners such as DTx, assuming they have demonstrated that they are safe and effective to be used by our clinicians and patients, starts with a discussion about data. It's important for us to understand the data sources—type and quality of the data sources that have been used to feed and train the model, the context these data have been derived from, and would it be applicable to our local context here, at the hospitals where the technology might be deployed and used." Read more from Dr. Ngiam on best data practices for implementation in chapter 9.

Similarly, to ensure the integrity of any data-driven initiative, it is crucial that the data in question are legally sourced. Data provenance—the records on how and where the data were collected and what has happened to them since—inform to a great degree the quality, authenticity, and credibility of the data. These factors substantially influence everything from the adequate training and external validation of AI algorithms to how patients can be stratified for treatment, among other critically important parameters. Importantly, datasets can also serve as a source of bias, a major challenge that can adversely impact the health outcomes of patients who were underrepresented in the datasets, for example patients with rare medical histories, or patients from low- and middle-income countries. Bias—a systematic error in preference of an idea vs. its alternative—is present in both human and algorithmic decision-making. Bias in medicine has a far-reaching consequence on the individual and population health outcomes.

The first step in overcoming biased decision-making is the understanding of where it is coming from. In case of the algorithmic decision-making, the first place to check for bias is the underlying data used by the algorithm. A reliable and trusted data source does not guarantee the data's relevance to the population you are trying to help. For example, a dataset of otherwise good technical quality (i.e., consisting of thousands of patients, well organized, traceable, and with an acceptable level of missing data fields) but in which the average member is a 55-year-old white male with a body mass index (BMI) of 35 can lead to a biased interpretation of an average diabetes patient's clinical profile and influence the training data used in the development of the algorithm of a hypothetical DTx solution for diabetes. As a result, an algorithm built on such data may trigger automated insulin release at a dosage calibrated based on recommendations for a person with this particular physiological profile, and that could have serious implications if the same dosing were applied for a 21-year-old Asian female with a BMI of 18. To add even more complexity to the dosing problem, optimized insulin dosing parameters for certain patients may be highly individualized and not be directly correlated to traditional considerations such as body weight and/or BMI. In this scenario, an insulin overdose for the younger female could lead to hypoglycemia—a glucose level that is too low—with potentially serious outcomes, including loss of consciousness in extreme cases.

If an analytical tool is developed based on data from a clinical trial that used excessively rigorous inclusion and exclusion criteria, whereby only "ideal" patients were recruited (that is, people with no comorbidities), it may have limited application to patients in real-world situations, where disease symptoms may be less clear-cut and one's clinical biomarkers may reflect the impact of several intertwined health conditions. To avoid such missteps, the datasets used for developing, training, and validating algorithms, such as those that underpin DTx technologies, should represent patient populations that are as similar as possible to the ones the solutions intend to serve. And even then, one should keep in mind that data are not the only source of bias. The analytical tools, if incorrectly designed, can skew the decision based on the otherwise representative data. This can occur, for example, by applying a higher importance to predefined, biased factors. Being aware of the existence and risk of biases, in both datasets and the algorithms themselves, allows developers to incorporate design features that can limit them (e.g., fairness-aware machine learning) and for the overseeing body to put in place an appropriate framework to monitor and minimize any potential bias.

Who Owns the Data Processing Product?

The crowning achievement of your work is the product of your data processing. Collecting data can take years and requires a considerable investment in infrastructure and a skilled workforce, hence the options we presented to you on where you can find ready-to-use datasets. Once you have identified and gained access to the optimal data, you can use it to develop, validate, and refine your tool. At one point you will start collecting the data yourself and may even start forgetting about the challenges of your early search for the optimal dataset. Before that happens, though, there is an important question to be answered: who owns the product of your work given that all of the data upon which it is based has been laboriously collected by someone else from yet another party (the patient)?

The complexity of this question increases as the number of parties involved that contribute either data or design and technological know-how, or both, grows. "It is never too early to have a conversation with your business partners and collaborators about the ownership of the data and the data processing products," says our contributor Dr. Georgios Kaissis, senior research scientist at the Institute of Artificial Intelligence in Medicine and Healthcare and leader of the health care and research units at OpenMined, an open-source community developing privacy-preserving machine learning tools and training.[2] This conversation may not be easy, and it is helpful to refer to legal frameworks if they exist. Most common, the intellectual property (IP) rights—including the ownership of your DPP—may have to be specified on a case-by-case basis.

Nicholas Brocklebank, director of in-house legal digitization and transformation at the Global Legal Solutions Group, a provider of legal operations solutions and dedicated services for startups and the management of IP, points out that datasets are generally considered to be the intellectual property of the party that created them. So, to gain access to such datasets, you will require a license from that owner, the terms of which will be whatever you can commercially agree on with that owner.

What does this mean in practice? While some medical and research institutions charge a nominal fee, or no fee at all, for access to their data as part of their mission to support medical technology development, the parties owning the data are free to set any price they consider appropriate. It is not uncommon to see some organizations require either costly payments for access or ownership rights in any DPP that is developed with use of their data. Brocklebank tells us,

> The key to avoiding unpleasant surprises is to read the terms of any license agreement in detail before proceeding to access the dataset (easier said than done, as so many of us are used to clicking through stuff online, but this is really important). The upside of carefully reading license agreements is that if you consider the cost or terms to be excessive, but you still find the data valuable for your project, you can try to negotiate by reaching out to the data

owner—or simply look elsewhere for a similar dataset with more favorable access terms.[3]

Lastly, if the resulting technology is to be commercialized and monetized once it has been developed based on the licensed data, the parties will have to agree on profit sharing. It can get complex quite quickly if the project involves multiple parties providing data and/or technical developments. "One possible approach is to implement an infrastructure that tracks what data were used and what code was developed by each team so as to evaluate the contributions of each party, considering both quantity and quality," shares Dr. Kaissis. It may sound like a hassle, but with the global DTx market projected to reach US$11.82 billion by 2027, it is imperative to treat the ethical, legal, and technical foundations of this thriving ecosystem with the highest attention to detail.[4]

Data Privacy and Safety

With an increase in the digital literacy of current and future technology consumers, the user of digital technologies has a growing awareness of the value of their data and the threats related to data breaches. The demand for the increased control over one's data access has been heard by the regulators and by the tech companies. In 2018 the European Union established its comprehensive privacy protection law, known as the General Data Protection Regulation, signaling a readiness on the part of national and international regulators to step in and demand an increased control of data privacy and anonymity. Shortly thereafter, in 2019, the *New York Times* released a collection of articles on privacy titled The Privacy Project that featured an opinion piece by Google CEO Sundar Pichai ("Privacy Should Not Be a Luxury Good") in which Pichai outlined Google's strategies for data management that increased privacy.[5] Another technology giant, Apple, used privacy as a selling point for its iPhone 12 ad campaign highlighting the iPhone's App Tracking Transparency feature to manage data access when using the phone.

The desire for privacy (or the fear of losing it) can have real implications for the adoption of health care solutions, even if these solutions have a huge potential benefit. A good example of this scenario has been the reluctance of the general public to install COVID-19 contact tracing apps, as shown by a previous study assessing populations in Australia, France, and the United States.[6] Importantly, privacy concerns are only increasing and its consideration in the development and downstream use in DTx will need to be continuously addressed.

What does this mean for your DTx endeavor? Understanding privacy expectations and designing your product with built-in privacy protection mechanisms will help you not only avoid security and regulatory missteps but also minimize the risk of nonadoption and avoid issues of noncompliance down the line. To do this right, we recommend engaging a cybersecurity or privacy expert as soon as your technology passes the initial data collection, algorithm training, and validation stages. Here we highlight several high-level considerations for DTx platform deployment into the real world.

Privacy Threats

A key first step toward protecting privacy by design is identifying the threats. "Even if you have the best intentions in mind, if the data is attractive, it is under threat," says Professor Reza Shokri, a researcher of data privacy and trustworthy machine learning from National University of Singapore's School of Computing. The risk of privacy threats can be divided into direct and indirect information leakages. Direct information leakage occurs within an organization, for example, by breaking contextual integrity (using the data for a different application than what the data donor consented to). Indirect data leakage occurs when, based on the DPP or on data introduced into the system with an adversarial objective, one can reconstruct and deidentify the underlying dataset.

The Threat of Reidentification

There is a common belief that removing key identifiers, such as a person's name or identification number, is sufficient to ensure privacy. Unfortunately, this step is far from sufficient. Even more unfortunate is the fact that it may not guarantee protecting against patient identification, especially when those data are of value. However, knowing full well that more steps beyond removing key identifiers may be needed to effectively prevent patient reidentification, this may lead to questions of whether or not the resulting dataset will become so redacted that it is no longer useful.

One may also wonder how it is possible that data contributed by one individual cannot "hide" in the tens of thousands of other data points to naturally protect against reidentification. The explanation is that while a single attribute, such as gender or location, is not a key identifier and typically cannot be traced to a particular person, multiple attributes across high-dimensional datasets that are associated with the same person, such as gender, age, and multiple check-in locations, can be easily triaged by a skilled malevolent agent to reidentify that individual. These points illustrate why the issue of data security will always serve as a major consideration for companies in the digital health space.

Want to Go Further?

Data security and privacy preservation are rapidly and dynamically evolving fields. As the scholarly publications on these topics are frequently updated, we recommend following the work and educational resources of open-source communities, such as OpenMined, and leading organizations in the field, such as the Simons Institute at the University of California, Berkeley. It may also be helpful to explore the latest updates at key scientific and industry meetings, such as the Healthcare Information and Management Systems Society Global Health Conference, the Conference on Neural Information Processing Systems, and the Conference on Computer and Communications Security, among others.

Tools to Provide Data Safety

Direct information leakages can potentially be avoided by continuous evaluation and reevaluation of the strategies being employed by an organization to protect its data infrastructure. This can be further bolstered by robust auditing processes to assess the data-access workstreams within an organization, and this oversight applies to both raw and processed data. To address reidentification and other forms of indirect information leakage, various approaches and tools are being developed to ensure that both data processing and results publishing are done with safety features that protect the privacy of the individuals who have contributed their data. Some of those tools can be implemented at the level of your DTx platform, while others require buy-in from the broader community and the stakeholders with whom you want your technology to interface (e.g., a hospital or a health care system).

As in many other fields, data are a critical component of the validation of eventual deployment of medical innovation. For that reason, data should be viewed as both a vital business asset as well as highly sensitive personal information, provided by patients and users for the benefit of the global community. Responsible data sourcing and management entails safety, ethical, and legal compliance, and the principles of responsible data management should be integrated into emerging DTx platforms at the very start of their life cycles.

Key Takeaways

1. Datasets can be obtained from a range of sources. Whichever source or sources you choose to drive the development of your DTx platform should be carefully vetted since it will form the foundation of your innovation.

2. Data ownership and rights to the data processing product must be considered as early as possible in the innovation road map.

3. Privacy preservation is a critical consideration from ethical, legal, and adoption standpoints. Invest your time in implementing data management framework(s) that are appropriate and adaptive toward evolving needs and standards in data security and privacy protection.

NOTES

1. National University Health System, one of the three public health care clusters in Singapore, is composed of several hospitals, national specialty centers, and polyclinics. More from Dr. Ngiam on the stakeholder expectation can be found in chapter 9.

2. From an interview with the authors, December 10, 2020.

3. From an interview with the authors, January 12, 2020.

4. Precedence Research, "Digital Therapeutics Market Size to Hit US$ 11.82 Bn by 2027."

5. Pichai, "Privacy Should Not Be a Luxury Good."

6. Chan and Saqib, "Privacy Concerns Can Explain Unwillingness to Download and Use Contact Tracing Apps when COVID-19 Concerns Are High."

Clinical Validation

Unique Challenges and Novel Approaches

This chapter was coauthored with Jennifer Shannon, MD, CEO at Digital Brain Consulting, clinical advisor to several digital therapeutic companies, Regional Medical Director at Cognoa, and a member of the Digital Therapeutics Alliance Advisory Board; as well as Xavier Tadeo, PhD, clinical trial and regulatory affairs specialist at the N.1 Institute for Health at the National University of Singapore.

Digital therapeutics, like drugs, need to be established as being safe and effective. And much like the work that goes into bringing new medicines to market, supporting these objectives requires marshaling scientific evidence that attests to the clinical validity of these technologies.

First, the DTx must be validated using randomized controlled trials (RCT). Other research modalities commonly used for testing DTx are observational studies (where the researcher observes processes and outcomes without intervening or assigning treatments, and the results can be descriptive or analytical), real-world outcomes studies (research comprising real-world data to assess health outcomes and advise health care management), real-world evidence studies (analysis of real-world data obtained from retrospective or prospective observational studies), and economic evaluation studies (analysis of financial impact on the patient and payer via cost effectiveness analysis). These forms of analyses include considerations of quality-adjusted life year (QALY), or the cost to prolong life while accounting for the quality of life. Additional analyses may look at the equal value of life years gained (evLYG), which primarily assesses the degree to which life is lengthened irrespective of the quality of life gained. These strategies have served as pillars for how interventions can be assessed when their deployment is being considered.[1] Importantly, as the application of DTx continues to expand for such domains as chronic disease prevention and management, oncology, and other indications that generate substantial cost burden on health care systems and patients, the aforementioned measures represent both standards and calls to action to which DTx platforms have the opportunity to meet.

Studies that involve any identifiable health information or human biological material or that subject an individual to any intervention must be carried out under the supervision of an institutional review board (IRB) or other applicable institutional ethics/medical board and, in many cases, accompanied by a recommended listing on a publicly available registry, such as ClinicalTrials.gov or clinicaltrialsregister.eu, upon study launch. After the product is granted market access, evidence must still be collected and analyzed on an ongoing basis to support the product's effectiveness and safety assurances in a real-world setting and to possibly give insight into new, optimized iterations of the product. In a nutshell, if you are a DTx developer or entrepreneur, there are substantial bars to meet before a product can be considered for regulatory clearance, subsequent clinical deployment, and receipt of reimbursement codes from insurers where applicable.

With the emergence of digital health in the marketplace, there has been a corresponding increase in industry-academic partnerships to drive evidence generation. As with traditional research and development (R&D), DTx developers can and should collaborate with academic research centers and hospitals to facilitate and potentially accelerate many of the clinical and regulatory requirements for DTx commercialization. Some of the key advantages at the foundation of these partnerships include the ability to integrate the go-to-market framework of an industry-developed DTx with the rigor associated with IRB review and approvals, potential for collaborative clinical trial design and biostatistical method innovation, and ultimately, the codevelopment of peer-reviewed publications that serve as a bedrock for due diligence and independent evaluation of research evidence. Contract research organizations (CROs) can provide similar services, and partnering with them can be particularly useful in setting up multisite trial recruitment since data monitoring from numerous sites can be insurmountably challenging to manage without substantial infrastructure familiar with the regulatory environment in place. In addition, CROs can provide instrumental insight in later stages of the clinical validation of a DTx, when other stakeholders beyond trial participants are engaged.

Besides being established as effective for patients (users), and complying with legal requirements as well as ethical considerations, the clinical validation of a DTx represents a major inflection point when it comes to convincing potential investors to back a venture. Without validation, apps are subject to classification within the wellness category, an overcrowded space where standing out is a challenge. However, validation is expensive. To solve this paradox, entrepreneurs can potentially turn to grants and angel investors during certain stages of development prior to exploring the venture capital route.

Regardless of the funding route taken, investors and some grantors will require varying degrees of assurances, objectives, or other types of key performance indicators. Value metrics, such as the ones provided by the leading professional society for health economics and outcomes research (the International Society for Pharmacoeconomics and Outcomes Research, or ISPOR),[2] can help decision-makers to understand hard-to-measure benefits and costs (economical and clinical) of a therapeutic intervention.

The journey to DTx clinical validation presents some unique challenges not found in the traditional R&D process. Here we review eight of them in detail.

Defining Digital Clinical Endpoints

Clinical endpoints are assessment criteria that measure the safety, efficacy, and overall effect of an intervention (e.g., drug or therapy) in a clinical trial. These can refer to survival rates, occurrence of disease, biomarkers, evolution of symptoms, or drug toxicity, just to name a few. The five-year survival rate of stage IV cancer patients, decreases in viral load, and the frequency and severity of adverse events are some examples of clinical endpoints.

Digital endpoints, also known as digital biomarkers, are a subtype of clinical endpoints based on physiological and behavioral data tracked and measured digitally, often by the investigational device itself. Devices that collect highly accurate data from which such endpoints can be derived include accelerometers, activity monitors (also known as fitness trackers), digitally embedded microphones, and blood pressure sensors, to name a few. Examples of digital endpoints include heart rate, breathing rate, blood oxygen saturation, changes in speech patterns, or sleep duration and quality.

The unique value of digital endpoints for research is that they may augment the quality, quantity, and granularity of data collected in a trial. Because they typically do not require physical measurements by a nurse or a nurse technician and reduce the need for in-person visits to clinical study sites, they are likely to make clinical trials in which they are incorporated more attractive for potential participants. In effect, these trial designs and associated technologies can decentralize clinical trial execution, where participants are monitored remotely through automated dataflow. This approach has seen a substantial increase following the emergence of COVID-19. These decentralized trials in turn may drive patient enrollment and adherence, benefiting both patients and clinicians by freeing up time and eliminating trips and interactions that are not absolutely necessary. Indeed, in decentralized or hybrid trials, digital endpoints are indispensable, particularly when trial participants hail from rural areas or other low population density settings. These designs can dramatically advance observational and longitudinal studies by collecting data over time with markedly reduced workload and personnel required compared to traditional approaches. This in turn makes them an ideal instrument for the collection of real-world data, such as those generated during phase IV (post-marketing) pharmacovigilance studies.

In terms of therapeutic areas, digital endpoints are most useful for investigating conditions where human supervision can be partially automated or where clinical judgment and shared decision-making can be supported by algorithmic analysis. Hypertension, diabetes, and more "subjective" disciplines, such as psychiatry and neurology (which are largely based on observational assessments) are a few examples of areas where the application of digital endpoints can improve the quality of patient monitoring.

Companies interested in leveraging digital clinical endpoints through technology face some important entry barriers, however. Firstly, any association between a digital biomarker and a specific condition must be backed by solid clinical evidence. A notable challenge in this instance is showing that changes in the digital biomarker correlate with disease state in patient clinical outcomes. In other words, output data from the DTx using a digital biomarker need to appropriately reflect the clinical concept of interest. Moreover, the accuracy and reliability of digital biomarkers needs to be assessed against current standard biomarkers before regulatory approval; output data from the DTx using a digital biomarker needs to be accurate when compared to a gold standard.

Digital endpoints and biomarkers are relatively novel and a comprehensive regulatory framework that governs their adequate usage is yet to be developed. Thus, apart from developing, testing, and honing the hardware and software of their solution, DTx companies also need to establish and validate what they consider to be relevant endpoints for the therapeutic area in which they have chosen to operate.

In 2019 several pharmaceutical companies that sponsor clinical trials decided in the spirit of collaboration to share their intellectual property to create a public digital endpoint database, now available at the website of the nonprofit Digital Medicine Society (DiMe).[3] This database is applicable not only to DTx, but to all type of interventions whose effect is to be measured with digital biomarkers. This crowd-sourced resource allows such key stakeholders as principal investigators, DTx developers, and collaborating clinicians to search for standardized, validated clinical endpoints when developing digital health technologies. To cite one example, UCB Biopharma, a contributor to the DiMe database, shared the digital endpoints the company used in a phase IV trial to assess the efficacy of a wearable technology it had developed for improving patient adherence to the drug Neupro, commonly prescribed to mitigate Parkinson's disease symptoms.[4]

Meanwhile, for those who still prefer to develop their own digital biomarkers, the Clinical Trials Transformation Initiative (CTTI) has created recommendations and best practices for identifying, selecting, and developing novel clinical endpoints.[5] Cofounded by Duke University and the US Food and Drug Administration (FDA), CTTI is a group of more than 500 organizations devoted to driving the adoption of optimal trial design and execution practices to modernize research strategies among its community.

Comparing DTx to Standard of Care

Traditionally, randomized clinical trials follow a design where patients are allocated into one of two or more groups that can include control and treatment groups. Patients randomized into the control group receive either the standard of care or a placebo. As the standard of care is well defined,[6] this allows the experimental treatment to be compared to the control group in order to assess its relative efficacy and safety. To simplify, a hypothetical malaria patient randomized into a clinical trial for a new treatment and allocated to the control group could potentially receive the standard of care of chloroquine; a malaria patient allocated to the experimental group would be given the experimental drug. Alternatively, if ethical considerations allow it and withholding a standard of care treatment for the duration of the trial is not considered potentially damaging to the person's health, participants in the control group may also be "treated" with a placebo. In drug trials, this pill does not contain an active ingredient (a "sugar pill").

It should be noted, however, that the standard of care is hard to define for certain conditions that are usually the target of DTx (e.g., behavioral conditions). This may require additional considerations when the process of defining the value proposition of the DTx, where stakeholders and regulators will require an outcome improvement over the standard of care. Researchers can address these considerations by designing multiarm trials where one group receives the DTx intervention added to a given standard of care assessed against the standard of care alone.

Another way to address these considerations is to use as a control a digital placebo or a waitlist. This is often possible when evaluating digital interventions that address mental health in patients that have yet to receive treatment in a conventional setting. Suitable digital placebos are based on and delivered through an existing app framework, whereby the actual experimental intervention is replaced with generic information about the patient's condition, a game, or a mock treatment. A good example of a DTx solution that was developed and validated using alternative controls is EndeavorRX, formerly Project Evo, Akili Interactive's gamified DTx solution for the treatment of attention deficit hyperactivity disorder (ADHD). Evo harnesses a video game–based approach with increasing levels of distractions and difficulty but is carefully designed to target specific brain regions and improve cognitive function. In the clinical validation stage, Evo's developers created a digital placebo, also a video game (Boggle), where the patient would put together words from a set of letters. This placebo did not mediate effects on the ADHD condition of the patients while requiring the same duration of screen time as the Evo intervention. Sleepio, a DTx solution for the treatment of insomnia via digital cognitive behavioral therapy, is another digital health technology that created a digital placebo using the original platform and design but without the active therapeutic ingredient. A point to consider regarding the use of a digital placebo is controlling for any other factors that could impact improvement (e.g., placebo effect, effect of engagement with provider, or any other support that might come with the tool).

In addition to digital placebos, waitlist-based control groups receive treatment after the study and are a suitable alternative in cases when the participants' condition allows for a temporary delay in the treatment. Whether opting for either a digital placebo or a waitlist, however, researchers should expect an inflated effect size of the intervention being studied because of the effective absence of any treatment in the inactive comparator-based control arm. As the technology matures, too, it will give rise to opportunities for new versions of DTx to be tested against their predecessor or a competitor. In such cases, the "old" DTx could be used as an active comparator, although it may still not be recognized as the standard of care. Nonetheless, we expect that the standard of care landscape will change dramatically with the increasing adoption of DTx.

DTx Validation across Cultures and Stakeholders

DTx platforms able to successfully address their intended use while backed by clinical evidence at scale will ultimately transcend the boundaries of the country in which they were developed and first tested. As DTx platforms are eventually deployed across different cultural, national, and linguistic environments, important considerations pertaining to acceptance, uptake, and adoption may need to be addressed. While social differences might not be a challenge unique to DTx, they are a more prominent issue from a technology validation perspective than they are in the case of clinical research evaluating the effectiveness of a new drug or a physical device (e.g., an orthopedic brace). This is because DTx platforms target behavioral components, which may be closely related to societal norms and can therefore vary dramatically across cultures. DTx developers and researchers should take these differences into account when building their platforms, designing a trial, and mapping out implementation stages so that the outcomes reflect the true validity of the DTx when deployed in multicultural populations.

Likewise, emphasis should be placed on recruiting trial participants that reflect the diversity of the population in which the solution will be deployed.

Just as DTx designers and innovators need to account for diverse and culturally unique user bases, they should also expect variability in their potential users' personal attitudes toward the use of DTx. This variability may stem from such factors as age, socioeconomic status, familiarity with technology, or personal preference. Hence, as promising as the technology may be, it will only be an effective solution if people actually use it. DTx organizations need to conduct the necessary target population research that provide the initial insights about the expected adoption of their proposal. One way to obtain this information is by designing DTx clinical trials that use mixed quantitative and qualitative methods so as to assess acceptability and route toward widespread adoptability alongside safety and efficacy.

We would like to take a moment here to emphasize the critical role qualitative researchers play in DTx development. As noted earlier in our discussion about the importance of having the right team, qualitative research professionals bring an essential skill set by using an ethnographic lens to design questionnaires, surveys, focus groups, and other methods that capture user engagement and identify potential shortcomings of a digital intervention from a usability standpoint. These qualitative research methods can also be used to assess the usability, acceptability, and likely adoption of the DTx by all relevant stakeholders (i.e., caregivers, clinicians, health insurance reimbursement leads). We will see later in chapter 10, "Supporting Adoption of DTx," the importance of having such data points early in the DTx development road map.

Clinical Validation Does Not Translate into Widespread Adoption

Regulatory approval alone may not be enough to convince providers, payers, and investors of your DTx solution's value. This is because the regulatory approval after clinical trials is based on how "capable" an intervention is in a controlled setting, which can ultimately differ from the real world. The measures used to reflect the performance of an investigational therapy in these different settings are known as *efficacy* and *effectiveness*, respectively.

Efficacy refers to the performance of a treatment under the controlled environment of a clinical trial, with strict criteria for the inclusion and exclusion of trial participants. For example, possessing certain comorbidities may preclude someone from participating in a clinical trial while many future patients, who will eventually undergo treatment with the intervention post-approval, may have those same comorbidities. Nonetheless, in order to assess an intervention from a trial perspective, the importance of inclusion and exclusion criteria is evident. Effectiveness, on the other hand, refers to the performance of that same treatment in the real world, where it may be prescribed to and used by patients who did not participate in the trial and who may have very different characteristics from those who did participate. Clinical trials conducive to market access measure efficacy, yet stakeholders demand both efficacy and effectiveness. Of course, DTx are subjected to clinical trials, an integral part of cementing clinical evidence for premarket submissions to regulatory bodies. But unlike traditional clinical trials, DTx technologies and devices are typically tested directly in the market, in real-world settings.

Provided that a DTx solution has received FDA marketing approval, the company that develops and commercializes it must continue to demonstrate its effectiveness in the post-approval period, commonly by conducting a phase IV trial. Of note, DTx trials and their inherent potential for decentralization may markedly expand the impact of their resulting datasets due to the capacity for increased frequency of longitudinal patient monitoring over traditional study designs and logistics, among other considerations.

As mentioned earlier, some countries are starting to lay the groundwork to expand DTx by developing guidelines that can potentially enable such technologies to gain a foothold in the market. The National Institute for Health and Care Excellence (NICE) in the United Kingdom, for example, has developed an evidence standards framework for digital health technologies in collaboration with NHS England, Public Health England, and MedCity, a not-for-profit cluster organization for the health and life sciences sector in the London area. The framework describes standards of evidence—clinical and economical—required for a DTx to be considered valuable for the health care system. It assists DTx developers to create a plan to fulfill these requirements and helps commissioners to decide on whether to contract a DTx.[7] In 2019, Germany's parliament passed the Digital Healthcare Act (*Digitale-Versorgung-Gesetz*, also referred to as the DVG), which regulates the reimbursement of DTx. Specifically, publicly insured patients (90% of the German population) gained coverage for Class I or Class IIa (low risk) software medical devices or stand-alone software purposed for disease diagnosis, monitoring, and treatment. The DVG has also enabled entrepreneurs to apply for preapproval through a fast-track process. Subsequently, during a 12-month in-market trial period, the digital solution is tested for efficacy.[8] In 2020, the National Cryptologic Center in Spain released a guide with best safety practices for health app developers, including minimum requisites for safe data treatment and storage.[9]

N-of-1 Trials

As we mentioned earlier, controlled clinical trials—and RCTs in particular—are considered the gold standard of realizing and validating evidence-based medicine. However, many would-be trial participants are often unable to participate in studies due to inclusion and exclusion criteria. Since trial findings are largely based on a treatment's population-wide effects instead of individual outcomes, this is likely an opportunity to further enhance treatment efficacy and even pinpoint more responders to treatment compared to outcomes from traditional trial designs. Additionally, although a lack of comprehensive data precludes reliably calculating average RCT costs, it is indisputable that conducting RCTs can be a very expensive process.[10]

By contrast, N-of-1 trials, as they are known in the clinical litera-ture, generate evidence for an individualized treatment effect. These are clinical studies involving only one participant, whereby that per-son typically undergoes control (e.g., placebo, no treatment, or active standard-of-care treatment) and experimental intervention phases, with adequate "washout" periods in between, defined as the time be-tween treatment periods. The intervention sequence can range from a simple AB format (where A = control, B = experimental) to more com-plex sequences (e.g., ABBA, ABABAB) that allow researchers to assess the treatment effect over time, accounting for what statisticians call random errors, such as intermittent symptoms or temporary habits or diets that may affect the outcome. Essentially, a longer sequence can help to discern whether the results are consistently due to the assigned treatment, whereas an AB sequence may make it more difficult to know whether they are due to the treatment or to an unrelated, confound-ing factor.

By design, N-of-1 trials are patient-centric. With each patient effec-tively serving as their own control while also being addressed with multiple interventional permutations, more information may be gleaned from each participant compared to traditional trial designs. Optimal study targets for this type of trial are progressive or chronic conditions that are characterized by frequent symptoms and for which a known and actionable biomarker exists. Although data collection can be done in multiple ways, the "bespoke" nature of individualized clin-ical trials makes them an ideal environment for the use of sensor-based wearables, which facilitate longitudinal, passive (i.e., without the pa-tient needing to actively answer any questionnaires, keep a diary, re-spond to a clinical trial nurse's questions, submit himself or herself the physical measurements, etc.) collection of outcome measurements, of-ten a core component of DTx technologies.

Additionally, because of their unique study protocols designed to suit individual participants with specific health conditions, N-of-1 trials can benefit from continuous iterative improvements to their underlying data analytics systems. These systems or algorithms, whose outputs can lead to more precise and timely diagnostics, prognosis prediction, and personalized care processes, are one of the main types of use cases for the application of artificial intelligence (AI) in the health care domain. (Read more about AI applications in appendix A.) By leveraging preexisting population or individual data, as well as prospectively acquired data that are calibrated to the patient under treatment, AI can uniquely advance the personalization at the foundation of N-of-1 trials. With this information, AI can also generate predictive models or particular profiles to provide personalized diagnosis and therapy, allowing trial designs that dynamically customize the intervention at a participant level. CURATE.AI is an example of how AI can be successfully integrated in such trials.

CURATE.AI: A "Small Data" AI Approach to N-of-1 Trials

It is common knowledge that patients vary from one another. However, it is also important to note that patients can vary from themselves during the course of treatment. While it is also common knowledge that therapies exhibiting efficacy in a patient at the start of treatment may lose efficacy over time, treatments that don't mediate efficacy at the outset can, in certain circumstances, be misperceived as ineffective for the patient under care. If they can be administered optimally (defined as delivering the right therapies at the right respective doses), however, they can be effective. Resolving the right drug and dose parameters to optimize treatment for each patient, and doing this in a longitudinal and dynamic manner can be insurmountable using traditional population-derived approaches. This is where CURATE.AI comes in.

Current drug dosing methods rely on institutional guidelines and experience-based decisions by clinicians, which can lead to underdosing or overdosing events and the associated reduced effect or toxicity, respectively. Common AI approaches to treatment optimization train an algorithm to find statistical patterns based on preexisting population data, and the identified pattern is then used to treat an individual based on their characteristics. This big data approach to AI has some challenges, however. For example, it often requires large and comprehensive datasets that are representative of the population. Also, this approach might be suboptimally suited to certain subpopulations with very specific health conditions or characteristics. And it is very resource-intensive.

By contrast, CURATE.AI is a small data[11] platform, operating based on a single individual's dataset. Using an AI-derived algorithm, CURATE.AI builds a profile for that individual that predicts that person's likely response to different drug doses. Using this information, CURATE.AI can dynamically adapt the treatment dose for the most optimal outcome for that person. CURATE.AI is indication-agnostic, meaning that it can be applied to virtually any condition where there is a known and quantifiable biomarker (e.g., tumor size reduction, cognitive improvement) that yields a dose-dependent response to changes in input (e.g., drug dose, cognitive therapy intensity).

An important advantage of CURATE.AI over traditional personalization methods is that it does not require large amounts of population data, and the user profiles it builds can be recalibrated in the event of physiological changes. CURATE.AI is a clinical decision support system handled by a team of scientists that analyze the data and provide recommendations to clinicians. It has been successfully applied to drug dose personalization in solid tumor, infectious diseases, and posttransplant immunosuppression trials, and it is being currently tested for its applicability to improving cognitive function in people recovering from brain tumor surgery.[12]

The CURATE.AI proof-of-concept study was conducted as a prospective randomized controlled pilot trial where eight liver transplant patients were administered the immunosuppressive drug tacrolimus. The posttransplant patients needed to maintain their tacrolimus levels within an individually assigned target range that avoided both toxicity events and transplant rejection. The researchers used individual data generated by standard-of-care dosing methods to calibrate patient-specific CURATE.AI profiles and then leveraged the profiles to guide patient dosing. Patients randomized into the CURATE.AI group had less variability in tacrolimus trough levels than standard-of-care control patients. Of note, CURATE.AI-treated patients were discharged, on average, nearly one month earlier compared to standard-of-care patients.

This pilot study exemplifies a significant series of N-of-1 where every patient received a different treatment recommended by the same principle (CURATE.AI) and served as an example of harnessing digital medicine to innovate both trial design and novel capabilities in personalized treatment. Several qualitative studies are being conducted in anticipation of the future deployment of CURATE.AI to gauge the thoughts and attitudes of medical professionals and students toward using an AI platform as an aide during their decision-making process. For more insights into the importance of this process, please see chapter 10 on how to support DTx adoption and gain clinical buy-in.

Institutional Review Boards and N-of-1 Trials

A critical step toward the initiation of an N-of-1 trial is the IRB review process. N-of-1 trials can have two main objectives: personalized treatment or generalizable knowledge. The IRB typically presents different requirements based on the main goal. In cases where the intended effect is to evaluate and adjust treatment in direct patient care, an IRB should be consulted to identify the procedures and compliance measures needed to initiate this form of care, as guidelines can vary substantially between institutions and jurisdictions. More commonly, however, N-of-1 trials aim to produce generalizable knowledge that could inform optimal treatment for individuals with similar characteristics in the future. In these cases, the IRB may request that the study design be adapted to enable aggregated analysis of multiple identical N-of-1 trials.

CONSORT

To improve the reporting of RCT outcomes and to optimally communicate a trial's design, conduct, analysis and interpretation, the CONSORT (Consolidated Standards of Reporting Trials) Group launched the CONSORT 2010 Statement, an evidence-based guideline with a set of minimum recommendations to produce high-quality, standardized clinical evidence. Subsequently, the group developed the CONSORT extension for N-of-1 trials (CENT 2015), a framework to facilitate and standardize the reporting of N-of-1 trials.[13] The CENT 2015 guidelines highlight methodological considerations that differ from traditional clinical trial designs, such as statistical analysis, ancillary analysis, and outcome reporting. This framework also opens a critically important pathway toward realizing additional impact from N-of-1 trials. Specifically, adherence to such reporting guidelines allow for aggregated analysis of results from similar studies to provide further generalizable conclusions.

In summary, well-designed N-of-1 trials can serve as a pathway toward practice-defining evidence for individualized treatments. As such, they are well suited for testing DTx, which are highly customizable by nature due to the immense volumes of personal data they are designed and engineered to gather. In this context, the importance of AI is only expected to grow as it can tap into individual behaviors registered in a DTx, analyze the data and specific needs of a subject, and develop a targeted and potentially dynamically modulated intervention strategy.

Decentralized Clinical Trials

Digital health technologies leverage computing platforms, software, sensors, and telecommunications for health care uses, allowing the development of mobile health-compatible wellness and DTx apps. These technologies have enormous potential to give rise to new paradigms of remote clinical validation as well as downstream health care delivery, patient monitoring, and broader care-at-home workflows. There have been several denominations for these trials where mobile technology and decentralization converge: remote, virtual, siteless, digital, federated, and direct-to-patient are some of the names used by different groups, sometimes with disparate definitions for the same name. The most widely accepted denomination is the decentralized clinical trial (DCT). DCTs are described as trials executed through telemedicine and mobile/local health care providers, using processes and technologies differing from the traditional clinical trial model.[14] Similarly, remote decentralized clinical trials (RDCTs) have been defined as "an operational strategy for technology-enhanced clinical trials that are more accessible to [participants] by moving clinical trial activities to more local settings."[15]

DCTs utilize mobile technology and local health care providers, eliminating the need for substantial centralized infrastructure comprised of staff, investigators, and vendors across potentially multiple trial sites. There are many possible partial centralization options to apply depending on patient needs and the specific characteristics of the study; these configurations are adopted in so-called hybrid trials.

DCTs enable clinical trial teams to collect data directly from participants, without requiring in-facility visits. Even passive data collection without any direct information of the participant may be possible. These logistical considerations may allow for more convenient, patient-centric trials. With home-based participation, patient engagement may increase in all phases. Importantly, participant recruitment numbers may be higher, and therapy adherence, where applicable, may be aided for the participant. In summary, well-designed DCTs can improve data collection, data quality, and patient monitoring compared to traditional approaches. With DCTs, trial costs may be substantially reduced and timelines may be accelerated compared to traditionally conducted clinical research. Furthermore, data acquired from scenarios that resemble care at home may mirror real-world outcomes more effectively than clinically acquired findings, potentially better informing eventual consumer use considerations. The scattered territorial distribution of participants may also contribute to this effect by increasing biological and cultural diversity.

When designing DCTs or hybrid trials, it is important to consider trial, patient, and disease specificities to assess the optimal degree of decentralization (or the idea of decentralizing at all). Key questions include:

- Are there any assessments that need to be done in a clinical site?
- What is the geographical distribution of potential trial participants (e.g, rare disease patients may be more dispersed)?

- What are the local regulations regarding obtaining informed consent, remote interventions, and data collection?
- Is the device appropriate for independent use by patients less used to digital technology?

Additionally, many patients regard human connection among the most important aspects in the clinical trial experience.[16] Researchers will need to find the appropriate balance that allows patients some degree of in-person interaction with the clinical team but also the freedom to benefit from and contribute meaningfully to a trial remotely.

Several other challenges of DCTs are worth mentioning. In a DCT, patient authentication (e.g., verifying that a sensor is being worn by the participant) will be less straightforward than in a traditional trial. Ideally, measures should be in place to minimize these occurrences, and leveraging technology for authentication will be increasingly common (e.g., facial or other biometric identifiers).

Patient engagement with the intervention might, in some cases, decrease due to the decentralized design. As explained earlier, some individuals may prefer face-to-face interaction to feel involved in the intervention/treatment process. A hybrid approach that meets a broader spectrum of patient needs may in this case be an optimal and truly patient-centric approach. However, researchers should ensure that the data captured in different settings are comparable.

Regulatory authorities like the FDA and the European Medicines Agency have signaled that they are supportive of decentralized trials and are currently developing regulatory frameworks to modernize DCT oversight and ensure data leveraged from these trials are handled using transparent data standards.[17] Moreover, the CTTI has issued legal, regulatory, and practical recommendations on the adoption of decentralized clinical trials.[18] It is a deliberative process, boosted by the appearance of COVID-19 and the disruption the pandemic has caused in the execution of trials across the world, that will likely culminate in the alignment of international regulatory bodies in this respect and a potential mainstreaming of DCTs.[19]

Connected Clinical Trials

Despite digital health technology advancements, clinical trials are still by and large conducted the old-fashioned analog way. Current manual processes, such as data tracking and supply management, are error-prone and slow, while deficient patient monitoring and communication can increase patient risk. Adapting clinical trial infrastructure so that it integrates new technologies would increase trial efficiency, flexibility in the configuration of different trial aspects, and data security.

Realizing the power of digital solutions to optimize clinical trial efficiency and compliance, Tata Consultancy Services and Janssen Research & Development jointly built Connected Clinical Trials (CCT), a module-based platform for the digitalization and unification of all aspects of a trial. The module's eTracking feature facilitates registering and following the kits that are sent to participants; eLabel provides patient-specific electronic drug labels; eCommunication enables customized, real-time notifications; and eAdherence verifies medication intake thanks to smart blister packs that leave a time stamp when a pill is extracted, potentially allowing clinical trial staff-initiated intervention to improve timely dosing. Data collected through these features will subsequently be analyzed and sent to the relevant team members.

A phase I technical trial to assess the CCT platform was carried out with healthy subjects to test integration, communication, and user satisfaction. Trial participants were provided with smart blister packs containing placebo and a smartphone where they could download the study app. The results showed strong compliance and high acceptance of electronic labels, smartphone functions, and data uploading by patients, and demonstrated the potential to eliminate or reduce the use of paper and associated data-entry errors, improve the experience of trial staff, and obtain real-time insights to strengthen treatment safety.

Challenges with DTx Data Analysis, Sharing, and Storage

Most clinical trial data are collected directly from the patient. When this collection is done digitally, it is usually done passively, but digital technologies can generate much higher volumes of data in real time with superior accuracy and frequency compared to traditional methods of data collection. Given this avalanche of data, automated AI-based analysis techniques, such as machine learning, can be used to monitor, analyze, predict, and detect trends and anomalies in these large datasets on an individual and population level. For physicians, the rapid identification of patterns and possible adverse events opens the door to advancing dynamically personalized care into clinical practice, and it can ultimately lead to improved outcomes for their patients or, if used as a screening tool, reveal early signs of disease in the target population. In their most advanced form, machine-learning algorithms also make it possible for DTx technologies to learn by continuously streaming and updating user data and adjusting outputs. This increasing complexity of information flow, potential for automation, and potential ability to dynamically evolve the treatment approach represent a challenge for data analysis and regulation.

Data storage and sharing of a continually growing and changing dataset also present challenges, as current digital infrastructures are generally not adapted to store longitudinal data or to perform real-time analysis. Additional data storage and security infrastructures, data sharing agreements, and other factors surrounding compliant stewardship may need to be considered for dynamically evolving data repositories. Traditional electronic data capture forms are based on paper processes and cannot store different types of data in one place. As a result, electronic records may end up in separate repositories, hindering communication between stakeholders and systems (e.g., devices, researchers, vendors, sites, CROs, trial sponsors).

It is of paramount importance to acquire tools that integrate data management and collection from different sources and in nonconventional formats into a centralized resource. In recognition of this rapidly evolving space, regulatory agencies are starting to lay out a holistic framework to assess the pertinence of a DTx platform's access to market based on a number of factors. These include intended purpose, quality control mechanisms, level of human intervention, value added to the clinical workflow, risks and mitigation measures, and continuous learning plans and version controls for subsequent iterations of the DTx, among others. At the foundation of this infrastructure, all parties handling data should have aligned knowledge of the trial data flow and storage. To provide further insights into this important topic, CTTI's Mobile Technologies recommendations are a helpful resource in this respect.[20]

Deciding on the Optimal Regulatory Route

Due to the recent inception of the DTx space, guidance from the international regulatory community is still evolving. Generally, DTx regulatory approval or clearance requirements depend on the product claims regarding risk, efficacy, and intended use. Validation of efficacy and safety claims by regulatory or equivalent national bodies is required for DTx that treat or manage a disease, whereas for DTx platforms that claim to improve health function or prevent a disease, the degree of oversight may depend on additional factors outlined by local regulatory frameworks.[21]

In the United States, DTx platforms are regulated by the software as a medical device (SaMD) framework developed by the International Medical Device Regulators Forum. Most of the platforms have been designated as Class II (moderate to high risk) or Class III (high risk) devices as per FDA classification. Market clearance can be obtained with a 510(k) premarket submission that demonstrates the device is substantially equivalent to a legally marketed device (called a predicate). This clearance—the usual route for Class II devices—avoids the need of a costly and lengthy clinical trial, as long as the sponsor, defined as the person or organization who takes responsibility for and initiates the clinical investigation, ensures compliance with applicable risk controls.[22]

If the FDA designates a device as not substantially equivalent to the predicate, or if there is no predicate, or the sponsor suspects the device would receive a Class III classification, a De Novo risk-based classification can be requested, which can assign to the device a lower risk classification. The De Novo route allows for the marketing of devices for which applicable risk controls provide reasonable assurance of safety and effectiveness for the intended use.[23]

Class III devices require premarket approval (PMA),[24] and to collect clinical data for the PMA, an investigational device exemption is required before using the device in a clinical trial and shipping it across state lines.[25] When possible, deciding between FDA clearance and approval should take into account what kind of evidence will be required by the sponsor's target stakeholders.

It is important to note that the same product can be subject to a different regulatory workflow, including no regulation at all, depending on the intended use claimed by the sponsor (e.g., wellness vs. diagnosis). In some cases, the sponsor will claim their product is a medical device, and the FDA will determine that the product is actually a device but will exercise "enforcement discretion" and not regulate it.[26] The FDA could also grant temporary market authorization for a DTx during the course of a public health emergency after an interactive review process culminates in an Emergency Use Authorization.

In the European Union, DTx platforms qualify as medical device software (MDSW) and are covered by the EU Medical Device Regulation, or Regulation (EU) 2017/745 (EU MDR).[27] MDSW is software intended to be used, alone or in combination, for a purpose as specified in the definition of medical device in the EU MDR. The EU MDR distinguishes Class I, IIa, IIb, and III devices, from low to high risk and low to high regulatory requirements. Rule 11 of the EU MDR states that software intended to provide information used to make decisions with diagnosis or therapeutic purposes belongs to Class IIa, except if those decisions may cause death or an irreversible health deterioration (Class III) or a serious health deterioration or a surgical intervention (Class IIb). Software intended to monitor physiological processes is classified as Class IIa, except for monitoring of vital physiological parameters, where parameter variation could cause immediate danger to the patient, in which case it is classified as Class IIb. Rule 22 of the EU MDR applies to active therapeutic software with an integrated diagnostic function that determines patient management and leads to Class III.[28] Consequently, DTx will fall into Class IIa or higher and will require a Certificate of Conformity by a Notified Body.[29]

In Singapore, the import, manufacture, export, and supply of medical devices is regulated by the Health Sciences Authority (HSA). In 2021, the agency issued a guidance document on the regulatory requirements of any software that falls under the medical device definition according to the Health Products Act. DTx sponsors must submit to HSA a premarket product registration application to prove they comply with the essential principles for safety and performance of medical devices. Clinical evidence requirements will depend on the purpose of the generated information (to treat or diagnose, to drive clinical management, or to inform clinical management) and the seriousness of the medical condition.

The fast-changing landscape of digital technologies is driving authorities to develop specific regulatory pathways. The FDA launched the Digital Health Software Precertification Program to streamline DTx submissions from manufacturers with accredited quality standards.[30] Also, the FDA's Center for Devices and Radiological Health released a product lifecycle–based regulatory framework for AI- and machine-learning-based SaMDs.[31] In the UK, as mentioned earlier, the NICE has developed an evidence standards framework for digital health technologies to help developers understand the clinical and economical evidence standards required for their product to be considered valuable for the health care system. For the latest regulations, DTx organizations should investigate their market-specific regulatory standards and requirements.

Conclusion

Developing a DTx solution requires the ability to prove its efficacy through clinical validation, which is a complex process. It requires the interdisciplinary efforts of engineers, ethicists, clinicians, and health care decision-makers to address DTx-specific challenges arising from the novelty and particular characteristics of digital interventions. Those same features, however, may allow for the downstream design of innovative, participant-centric trials where DTx are tested with unprecedented efficiency and objectivity. Regulatory bodies, agencies, and associations are addressing those specificities and paving the way for a more streamlined DTx validation process by creating guidelines, collaborative databases, and distinct pathways for approval.

Key Takeaways

- Clinical validation is a necessary step toward DTx market introduction, whereby safety and efficacy are assessed through established controlled trial design principles, often a randomized clinical trial (RCT).
- DTx clinical trials may employ digital endpoints (safety and efficacy assessment criteria that are digitally collected and analyzed) that increase the accuracy and objectivity of the final analysis, but which also need to be validated. The Digital Medicine (DiMe) website includes a collaboratively sourced database of validated digital endpoints.
- DTx trials can circumvent the absence of consensual standard of care with multiarm designs testing standard of care, standard of care plus DTx, and DTx alone.
- It is important for DTx platforms to be validated across cultures, demographics, and stakeholders through mixed quantitative-qualitative methods in order to realize broadly actionable insights into effectiveness and safety.
- DTx are well suited for N-of-1 trials, which provide the highest-grade evidence for individualized treatment effect.
- DTx trials may be easily adapted to decentralized and hybrid trial designs, which can improve recruitment, retention, and therapy adherence while reducing costs.
- DTx platforms can generate vast amounts of trial data that can in turn lead to substantially enhanced analytical insights compared to conventional trial designs, provided the right infrastructure is available.
- In the context of a digitally delivered therapeutic, real-world evidence can be equally or more relevant than controlled clinical trial outcomes.

NOTES

1. Institute for Clinical and Economic Review, "Cost-Effectiveness, the QALY, and the evLYG."

2. ISPOR, "About HEOR," accessed September 10, 2021, https://www.ispor.org /heor-resources/about-heor.

3. Digital Medicine Society, "DiMe's Library of Digital Endpoints, accessed September 10, 2021, https://www.dimesociety.org/index.php/knowledge-center /library-of-digital-endpoints.

4. UCB Biopharma, "Study to Evaluate the Impact of Using Wearable Devices in Addition to Standard Clinical Practice on Parkinson's Subject Symptoms Management."

5. Clinical Trials Transformation Initiative, *Developing Novel Endpoints Generated by Digital Health Technology for Use in Clinical Trials.*

6. Standard of care is "treatment that is accepted by medical experts as a proper treatment for a certain type of disease and that is widely used by healthcare professionals. Also called *best practice, standard medical care,* and *standard therapy*" (National Cancer Institute, *NCI Dictionary of Cancer Terms,* accessed September 10, 2021, https://www.cancer.gov/publications/dictionaries/cancer-terms/def/standard -of-care).

7. National Institute for Health and Care Excellence, *Evidence Standards Framework for Digital Health Technologies.*

8. Federal Ministry of Health, "Driving the Digital Transformation of Germany's Healthcare System for the Good of Patients: The Act to Improve Healthcare Provision through Digitalisation and Innovation (Digital Healthcare Act—DVG)."

9. Centro Criptológico Nacional [National Cryptologic Center], "Requisitos de seguridad para aplicaciones de cibersalud [Security Requirements for eHealth Applications]."

10. Speich et al., "Systematic Review on Costs and Resource Use of Randomized Clinical Trials Shows a Lack of Transparent and Comprehensive Data."

11. Small data are data of accessible volume and format for humans. The accepted definition says that "small data connects people with timely, meaningful insights (derived from big data and/or 'local' sources), organized and packaged— often visually—to be accessible, understandable, and actionable for everyday tasks" (Allen Bonde, "Defining Small Data," *Small Data Group* (blog), October 18, 2013, https://smalldatagroup.com/2013/10/18/defining-small-data). Although humanity has based most of its advancements on small data, the concept appeared recently in opposition to the ubiquitous big data, which are data too large or complex to understand or analyze by common means. Small data are cheaper, all around us, and can have many applications, especially in the health care and marketing fields (e.g., streamlining shopping, personalizing fitness routines, tracking habits, predicting behaviors).

12. Zarrinpar et al., "Individualizing Liver Transplant Immunosuppression Using a Phenotypic Personalized Medicine Platform"; Shen et al., "Harnessing Artificial Intelligence to Optimize Long-Term Maintenance Dosing for Antiretroviral-Naive

Adults with HIV-1 Infection"; Pantuck et al., "Modulating BET Bromodomain Inhibitor ZEN-3694 and Enzalutamide Combination Dosing in a Metastatic Prostate Cancer Patient Using CURATE.AI, an Artificial Intelligence Platform"; Kee et al., "Harnessing CURATE.AI as a Digital Therapeutics Platform by Identifying N-of-1 Learning Trajectory Profiles."

13. CONSORT, "N-of-1 Trials," accessed September 10, 2021, http://www.consort-statement.org/extensions?ContentWidgetId=47627.

14. Clinical Trials Transformation Initiative, *CTTI Recommendations: Decentralized Clinical Trials.*

15. Trials@Home, "About RDCT's," accessed April 10, 2023, https://trialsathome.com/about-rdcts.

16. Anderson, Borfitz, and Getz, "Global Public Attitudes about Clinical Research and Patient Experiences with Clinical Trials."

17. Gottlieb, "Breaking Down Barriers between Clinical Trials and Clinical Care."

18. Clinical Trials Transformation Initiative, *CTTI Recommendations.*

19. Byrne, "DIA 2021 Set to Shed Some Light on Decentralized Trials Process, Accelerated Approval Pathways."

20. Clinical Trials Transformation Initiative, *Digital Health Trials: Recommendations for Delivering an Investigational Product.*

21. Digital Therapeutics Alliance, "Understanding DTx."

22. US Food and Drug Administration, "Premarket Notification 510(k)."

23. US Food and Drug Administration, "De Novo Classification Request."

24. US Food and Drug Administration, "Premarket Approval (PMA)."

25. US Food and Drug Administration, "Investigational Device Exemption (IDE)."

26. Coravos et al., "Digital Medicine: A Primer on Measurement."

27. See https://eumdr.com for the latest on the European Union Medical Device Regulation.

28. EUR-Lex, Document 02017R0745-20170505, May 5, 2017, https://eur-lex.europa.eu/eli/reg/2017/745/2017-05-05.

29. European Commission, "Internal Market, Industry, Entrepreneurship, and SMEs: Conformity Assessment."

30. US Food and Drug Administration, "Digital Health Software Precertification (Pre-Cert) Pilot Program."

31. US Food and Drug Administration, "Artificial Intelligence and Machine Learning in Software as a Medical Device."

CHAPTER 8

Factors That Influence the Implementation of New Technologies

This chapter was cowritten with Dr. Robyn Mildon, Founding Executive Director of the Centre for Evidence and Implementation with offices in Australia, Singapore, and the United Kingdom. Dr. Mildon is an internationally recognized leader in the fields of implementation science, evidence synthesis, and knowledge translation, as well as policy evaluations in health, education, and human services.

DTx platforms are designed to induce cognitive, behavioral, and physiological changes. As such, their effectiveness can vary dramatically across clinics, demographic segments, and countries due to culture, religion, values, or social context. To add to this complexity, technological, legal, and organizational factors related to the wider ecosystem into which DTx are deployed may also influence their implementation. These factors greatly condition local adoption of a DTx and must therefore be carefully identified, analyzed, and considered both in the initial design and the subsequent iterations of the technology.

Numerous research studies have been done to characterize these factors. Resulting theories and models of technology adoption have been proposed that can help innovators predict the response of end users.

These include the theory of diffusion of innovation, the unified theory of acceptance, the task-technology fit model, the use of technology model, and the technology acceptance model.[1] These models define key factors that influence the adoption and use of technology, such as perceived ease of use of a technology, perceived usefulness, social impact, facilitating conditions, attitudes to use, and users' behavior.[2]

As the evidence on factors specifically and uniquely relevant to DTx adoption is still emerging, DTx organizations should learn from similar technologies being implemented in similar contexts. For example, e-health technologies, electronic medical records, and clinical decision support systems can serve as sources of learning.[3] In a recent systematic analysis of 44 reviews of e-health technology implementation, the authors identified 10 key factors that influenced successful implementation (table 8.1).

Table 8.1. Factors that influence the implementation of e-health technologies

Innovation characteristics	• Adaptability (of the technology to fit the local context) • Complexity (e.g., difficulty level of the hardware and software, slow system performance, connectivity issues, etc.) • Cost (of the technologies and those associated with their implementation)
Outer setting[1]	• External policy and incentives (absence or inadequacy of legislation and policies and liability concerns)
Inner setting[2]	• Implementation climate (compatibility or general fit between the technology intervention and the organization)
Individual characteristics	• Knowledge and beliefs (attitudes of practitioners toward the technology and beliefs about its potential benefits) • Other personal attributes (health care professionals' computer skills, abilities, and experience)
Process	• Planning (for implementation) • Engaging (i.e., designation of champions and engagement of key stakeholders) • Reflecting and evaluating (to ensure system benefits, to increase health professionals' acceptance through demonstration of benefits, and to secure ongoing funding)

Source: Jamie et al., "Factors That Influence the Implementation of e-Health."
[1] Outer setting refers to the economic, political, and social contexts where the organization resides (e.g., policies, financing, stakeholder relationships).
[2] Inner setting refers to the structural, political, and cultural contexts where the implementation takes place.

In another systematic review of studies looking at factors impacting clinicians' adoption of mHealth tools, as many as 55 technological, social, and organizational factors were identified.[4] This provides a sense of the complexity of implementing new technologies in health care.

Usability as a Factor of Influence

Let's consider usability (often associated with complexity) as a factor identified across many of these reviews to see how well existing digital health tools for diabetes management have integrated them into their design. We selected this therapeutic area as an example because usability has been shown to be an adoption barrier for patients with diabetes and physicians who treat such patients.[5]

Usability measures how well a specific user in a specific context can use a solution to achieve a defined goal effectively, efficiently, and satisfactorily. Conceptually, it is related to ease of use, which is the effort required to use a particular product, service, or technology. In a systematic literature review of the social, organizational, and technological factors impacting clinicians' adoption of mobile health, usability was identified as one of the crucial elements impacting one's intention to use such technologies, but usability alone was not enough for user acceptance.[6] Layout, interface, and culturally appropriate and patient-centered design were also seen as key influencing factors in several studies included in the review.

In another systematic review, when 66 diabetes mobile applications with usability as an evaluation factor were compared and graded on a 5-point scale, the average score was 3.3, with scores varying from 2.5 to 4.1. This assessment reflects a neutral (or average) expression of these solutions' usability. It was also found that only 8% of mobile applications for diabetes were sufficiently interoperable to enable connection to an external sensor or measuring device, such as a blood glucose monitor.[7] For innovation and business leaders focused on providing a seamless, satisfying user experience, a technology that leaves room for improvement in terms of usability will encounter challenges in being adopted. Patient-centered solutions, leading to better patient experience and therefore higher levels of user satisfaction, can result in better patient engagement. Therefore, it will be essential for DTx organizations to not only define what would be a "good enough" patient experience while using the DTx but also consider how this experience can catalyze sustained user engagement while ultimately facilitating widespread adoption.

A DTx solution through its design, features, and overall usability should connect with its users—patients, caregivers, and clinicians—on a functional and potentially emotional level as well. For example, more research and consideration are needed surrounding the challenges and attitudes elderly patients or individuals with cognitive impairment have with maneuvering digital apps. Insufficiently addressing these challenges may reduce the usability of the technology for those segments of the population. Therefore, it is critical to understand the needs and motivations of the target users of a given DTx solution in the context in which they intend to use it, as well as the interactions with the app that will be required of them to fulfill those needs.

Local Context Matters

To optimize the pathway to widespread adoption of a DTx platform, usability and other factors that influence the implementation of digital health technologies should be user-centric. We stress the importance for DTx innovators to deeply engage with the contextual phenomena that impact and interact with the heterogeneous needs at the individual user level, whether that be for patients, caregivers, or physicians, as well as the ability to answer the specificities of a local context. This is not a trivial task. Even established, multinational companies undertake substantial effort to understand how contextual factors impact technology implementation and adoption. These efforts can lead to important lessons learned and a wealth of knowledge that can help future entrepreneurs.

In 2018, Google deployed a deep learning program across 11 clinics throughout Thailand to screen for diabetic retinopathy (DR) and evaluate the performance of the algorithm in a real-world clinical setting. The system sought to improve clinical workflows and patient outcomes in a country with a shortage of ophthalmologists and where diagnosis and treatment of diabetic retinopathy can be strengthened by a more efficient health care service. The program established the importance of accounting for several socioenvironmental factors at the foundation of their solution for the local context, which were key drivers of technology performance and the clinical experience for both the patient and clinical team.[8] Let's explore in detail the four factors initially deemed to be critical to the success of Google's AI system and that have served as a valuable source of insight into factors that drive patient and provider adoption.

The Importance of Localization, Learnings from Google

With regard to technical performance, Google's AI system was impressive—it could detect referable cases of retinopathy with an accuracy of 90% using only the analysis of a single photo of a diabetic's retina.[9] The value proposition was simple—provide ophthalmologist-grade diagnostic capability at scale. The screenings didn't require ophthalmologists to be involved at all. The nurses simply needed to take photos of the retina and upload them into the Google's AI system, and within approximately 10 minutes the patient could expect a diagnosis. By comparison, the traditional process required sending the photos to ophthalmologists and took from 2 to 10 weeks to get back.

Google's AI-based screening system was a promising solution to the common problem of health care workforce shortages in low- and middle-income countries. Its deployment illuminated several key factors that are critical toward clinical utility and user adoption.

Factor #1. Presence of Consistent Workflow and Screening Conditions across Clinics

In an ideal health care system, clinical workflows and patient management protocols are well documented, consistent from clinic to clinic. During the deployment process, it was noted that there was a high degree of variation in the eye-screening process from clinic to clinic. This was driven by the large degree of autonomy given to the nurses to organize this process depending on resources available at the time and basic infrastructures at their disposition (e.g., only two clinics had a dedicated screening room).

As a result of this variability, approximately 80% of the submitted images fulfilled the AI model's quality requirements, which prolonged the nursing team workflow. The image variability resulted in the retake and resubmission of images, adding 2–4 minutes spent per patient while local protocols allocated 90 seconds per patient due to the high volume of patients requiring screening. This consideration revealed the importance of aligning technology execution with local workflow considerations.

Factor #2. Presence of a Reliable Network Connection

In a health care setting with a strong internet connection, image processing and display typically requires a few seconds. However, due to the local IT infrastructure, Google experienced slower and less reliable connections than anticipated. Some images took up to 60 seconds or even 90 seconds to upload, which slowed down the photo analysis process and lowered the number of patients that could be screened compared to original estimates.

Factor #3. Patients Embracing the Proposed Solution

When the technology and internet connection worked well, patients would have their diabetic retinopathy result within 10 minutes. Following a DR-positive diagnosis, and if acceptable images could not be obtained after several tries, the study protocol recommended that the nurse advise patients to see a specialist. In Thailand, however, a referral to a nearby hospital could mean driving up to one hour, repeated queuing, and additional costs to the patient, which represented a substantial burden for the patients. In one clinic, up to 50% of the patients elected not to join the study as they were not agreeable with this potential ophthalmologist referral, and the associated "risk" to travel. In this case, despite access to a powerful technology platform, the workflow and potential for additional referrals created a challenge for widespread adoption.

Factor #4. Nurses Embracing the Proposed Solution

A key aim of the AI-based retinopathy screening system was to optimize clinical workflows and reduce the nurses' workload. The AI screening system eliminated the need for the nurses to perform an initial grading of the severity of retinopathy and check for apparent abnormalities. In practice, while the solution shortened the workflow by one step, additional steps were added, and infrastructural challenges were illuminated during the trial process. Nonetheless, the Google team recognized that "formative research that provides a strong understanding of clinical users and their context is critically important to the success of such a system. By incorporating human-centered evaluations into deep-learning model evaluations, and studying model performance on live data generated at the clinical site, we can reduce the risk that deep learning systems will fail in the wild, and increase the likelihood for meaningful improvements to patients and clinicians."[10]

Conclusion

Google's study not only provided many important insights to their team but also serves as an example to the DTx community of some of key factors to consider when designing their implementation strategies. The success of health-related technologies does not rest solely on their technical accuracy; it also rests on their ability to fit into the deployment context to ultimately improve patient care.[11]

To ultimately change practice in medicine, any technology, including DTx, should be designed and implemented sustainably. Understanding the needs, attitudes, and behaviors of clinicians, health care consumers, family members, and policymakers (the latter because they influence the design of health systems in which interventions take place) in the context in which they work and live are key factors for the intelligent design and long-term adoption of DTx. In this process, DTx organizations can draw inspiration from mHealth tools and similar technologies to leverage their lessons learned on technology implementation in health care. Considerations include adopting a cocreation approach that engages all stakeholders early on. In the next chapter, we will take a deep dive into understanding clinicians' perspectives and using that understanding to drive the adoption and prescribing of DTx.

NOTES

1. Garavand et al., "Factors Influencing the Adoption of Health Information Technologies."
2. Garavand et al., "Factors Influencing the Adoption of Health Information Technologies."
3. Jacob, Sanchez-Vazquez, and Ivory, "Social, Organizational, and Technological Factors Impacting Clinicians' Adoption of Mobile Health Tools."
4. mHealth is a subcategory of e-health defined as "medical and public health practice supported by mobile devices, such as mobile phones, patient monitoring devices, personal digital assistants, and other wireless devices" (Jacob, Sanchez-Vazquez, and Ivory, "Social, Organizational, and Technological Factors Impacting Clinicians' Adoption of Mobile Health Tools").
5. Klonoff and Kerr, "Overcoming Barriers to Adoption of Digital Health Tools for Diabetes."
6. Jacob, Sanchez-Vazquez, and Ivory, "Social, Organizational, and Technological Factors Impacting Clinicians' Adoption of Mobile Health Tools."
7. Arnhold, Quade, and Kirch, "Mobile Applications for Diabetics."
8. Beede et al., "A Human-Centered Evaluation of a Deep Learning System Deployed in Clinics for the Detection of Diabetic Retinopathy."
9. Beede et al., "A Human-Centered Evaluation of a Deep Learning System."
10. Beede et al., "A Human-Centered Evaluation of a Deep Learning System," 10.
11. Shah, Milstein, and Bagley, "Making Machine Learning Models Clinically Useful."

Recommendations for DTx Implementation

The section in this chapter on addressing implementation traps was cowritten with Dr. Robyn Mildon, Founding Executive Director of the Centre for Evidence and Implementation. Dr. Mildon is an internationally recognized leader in the fields of implementation science, evidence synthesis, and knowledge translation, as well as in program and policy evaluations in health, education, and human services.

Following the identification of factors that may influence DTx implementation in health care settings, DTx inventors are approaching the implementation stage. At this point, health care organizations will carefully assess the potential of new technologies, including DTx, against the risk they pose to patients, physicians, clinical workflows, and the system's business model.

Medical technology innovation holds immense potential, but there may also be health risks requiring consideration. That is why running a risk-benefit analysis of adopting new technologies underpins much of the decision-making processes that occur in health care. Due to the stakes involved, however, the default attitude at the point of initial assessment is typically one of strong aversion to risk. While this may be perceived as a frustrating hurdle from the perspective of an emerging DTx startup, by understanding the responsibility health care system managers have in such evaluations and embedding in the design of the DTx the risk management measures that anticipate elevated scrutiny, the chances that it passes the initial due diligence steps will significantly improve.

For this reason, in this chapter we highlight the expectations of health care system managers when it comes to implementing DTx at their hospital or clinic. We also discuss some of the most common implementation pitfalls at this stage and how to avoid them with an appropriate implementation strategy.

What Health Care System Managers Expect

We have already discussed the importance of demonstrating clinical evidence that DTx technology works, as well as the other benefits that a DTx can provide to patients, caregivers, physicians, and the health system as a whole. As a result, we will not return to those critical points but instead focus on the perceived risks and must-haves for DTx platforms. For this segment, we spoke with Dr. Ngiam Kee Yuan, Group Chief Technology Officer of the Singapore National University Health System (NUHS),[1] a health care system decision-maker involved with the evaluation of digital technologies for potential integration. In our discussion, he mentioned four elements for evaluation when considering DTx for NUHS, serving as key insights for DTx innovators:

Data Provenance and Clinical Validation

In assessing a new DTx proposition, one of the key features health care system managers first look at is the provenance of the underlying data (see chapter 6). To assure that a solution is safe and effective for use by clinicians and patients, it is important for DTx innovators to demonstrate that the data sources at its foundation have been appropriately vetted. Specifically, the type and quality of the data that have been used to feed and train the tool, the context in which these data have been collected, and the applicability of the model to the setting where the technology might be deployed are essential to determining whether it warrants further evaluation.

Security and Privacy

Privacy and security of health-related data are a top-of-mind concern for health care system managers, and for good reason. In 2019, the American Medical Collection Agency filed for Chapter 11 protection after revealing it had suffered an eight-month data breach that affected up to 20 million patients and in which the stolen data had been advertised for sale in underground web forums. In addition, among the largest ever data breaches occurred when the records containing personally identifiable information of about 80 million customers and employees of Anthem Inc., the second-biggest health insurer in the United States, were infringed.[2] Hackers have also been known to interfere with remotely accessible implantable medical devices, insulin pumps, and other medical technologies. As the implementation of DTx platforms into health care systems will simultaneously involve the deployment of companion software, security against potential hackers will be a critically important consideration for health care system managers. Therefore, it is essential to be prepared to answer how the patient-generated data elicited and channeled by the DTx will be handled, stored, and shared.

There are several approaches to protecting DTx-collected data your technology should be designed to handle. They are centered around detecting, separating, and securely storing personal identifiers, compartmentalizing highly dimensional data, encrypting data transfer, and safely storing the entire resulting datasets. To inspire confidence on the part of health care system managers and users, one will have to incorporate the highest privacy and security standards and readiness to adopt the health care system's existing data governance standards.

Technology Interoperability

Integrating DTx into day-to-day clinical care requires thinking across multiple dimensions by understanding the perspective of each of the stakeholders involved: physicians, patients, and health care administrators. While physicians will rightfully scrutinize the clinical evidence behind the DTx and patients its effectiveness and ease-of-use, administrators will be particularly concerned about its deployment within existing infrastructure. The end goal is making care delivery more seamless (and safe), rather than adding a new layer of complexity to existing solutions that all too often are already working in silos. Standardized billing and product codes will be necessary for electronic prescribing procedures, in addition to security requirements. Overall, modifications in electronic health record (EHR) and workflow integration are complex, depending on how DTx will be reimbursed through the different distribution channels.

Continuous Evolution of DTx

The continuous integration, continuous delivery, and continuous deployment (referred to as CI/CD in technical shorthand) of DTx technologies is critical to their utility. These concepts refer to how DTx platforms learn from the data and feedback they collect over time in order to improve health outcomes through high-precision insights and by providing a seamless experience to clinicians and patients. They also refer to how DTx adapt to potential changes in the system within which they have been deployed. This is applicable to both software and hardware, such as being compatible with new versions or updates to a hospital's EHR system or to a patient's mobile device. This further extends to how DTx fit within new mobile devices and new functionalities as they are introduced, such as better cameras, improved processing systems, and 5G networks.

To help DTx innovators think through these factors, we invite them to consider the following data management and security checklist, drawn up in the form of questions. It is not exhaustive, as there are sure to be other important issues that come up during the technology development and implementation cycle, but it contains the essential questions entrepreneurs should be able to address in order for their product to have a chance of interfacing with an existing health care system:

- ❏ Is the way the patient-generated data are used, stored, and shared compliant with local regulatory, environmental, and security standards as well as compliant with the partnering health care organization's standards?
- ❏ Do you have best-in-class data governance, privacy, and security standards with a comprehensive risk mitigation framework, encompassing preventable security and privacy breaches, cybersecurity risks, and potential disruption of care?
- ❏ Is there ease of DTx deployment (i.e., integration and interoperability) with the partnering health care organization?
- ❏ Is your DTx's strategy not only safe but also scalable?

Risk concerns can be a hindrance to the adoption of DTx. Therefore, as regulation of DTx evolves over the coming months and years, with new regulatory pathways, governance structures, data infrastructures, and security protocols being established, it is necessary for DTx entrepreneurs to build a sound data stewardship and interfacing foundation for their technology. This means investing in data management and security on the one hand, and engaging early on with health care institutions' chief technology and information officers on the other to make sure any new digital technology is compatible with existing and planned systems and workflows.

Although a solid technical and safety foundation for DTx technology is important, it does not guarantee commercial success. To prevent DTx venture failure when moving from development to commercialization, there are a few implementation traps that DTx innovators should be aware of and must overcome if encountered.

Addressing the Implementation Traps

Many of the experts interviewed for this book converge with findings from the existing literature on digital health technologies on the view that there are four main reasons why some DTx ventures fail when moving from development to commercialization.

No implementation strategy. Implementation or integration of DTx in business-as-usual clinical practice should be regarded as a process, not an event. As such, it should be planned and executed methodically in stages rather than as a one-off launch (a concept some DTx entrepreneurs might be tempted to borrow from the pharmaceutical industry's marketing approach to introducing new drugs). Many DTx start-ups do not have an implementation strategy for their product and rely on the idea that they can just "roll it out."

Implementation complexity and replicability. There is no simple or universally replicable way of implementing change—such as a new DTx platform—at scale in a deeply complex environment such as health care. You have already witnessed how a technology, pathway, or an approach can perform well in one setting but poorly or not at all in a different context. Well-thought-out implementation strategies, therefore, typically have multiple components and are adaptable to local health contexts, which are inherently complex because of their multiple interacting levels (e.g., patients, providers, teams, service units) and vary widely from setting to setting.[3] It is therefore crucial to understand—both qualitatively and quantitatively—the barriers and facilitators to implementing DTx in different institutional, cultural, and economic environments, since these will understandably impact their adoption by individuals and organizations.[4] In short, local context matters, but it also limits the replicability of technology implementation.

Not having the right know-how. No matter how carefully an implementation strategy is designed and planned in advance, the experience of actual implementation often generates novel or even unexpected insights that can improve the strategy "on the go" and in real time. Yet not all DTx startups have the necessary engine with the right team and know-how, training, or (importantly) adaptive mindset to use what is known in business innovation as the rapid cycle change model, an evolving implementation strategy to drive the spread of an innovation with some potential to adapt to different contexts.

All of these points are central to the implementation science (IS) approach that we introduced in our Part III introduction. To avoid falling victim to these implementation traps, DTx designers must think flexibly, understand local contexts, use qualitative methods to explore accepted processes and mechanisms, and be ready to adapt their intervention to achieve the best fit within different settings.

When developing, deploying, and evaluating a solution across multiple sites, we recommend that innovators have an implementation strategy based on a structured and phased approach. In short, follow an IS approach. It starts with having a clear definition of the proposed intervention and a plan for optimizing the components it consists of and the factors that influence its success. Ideally, that plan should be aligned with the evidence based on behavior change and tested through a series of small-scale trials in selected settings or through a rapid cycle test of the envisioned change model—in this case related to effecting behavioral change (figure 9.1).

The central element of the rapid cycle testing approach is the plan-do-study-act (PDSA) scientific method for testing a change by planning it, trying it, observing the results, and acting on what is learned. It ensures that ideas for change are tested and adapted for local contexts while paying explicit attention to opportunities for iterative improvement.

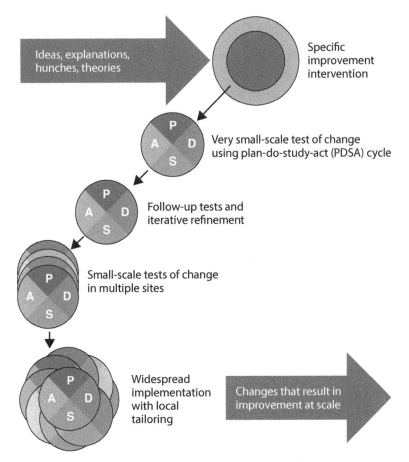

Ideas, explanations, hunches, theories

Specific improvement intervention

Very small-scale test of change using plan-do-study-act (PDSA) cycle

Follow-up tests and iterative refinement

Small-scale tests of change in multiple sites

Widespread implementation with local tailoring

Changes that result in improvement at scale

FIGURE 9.1. Rapid cycle test of a change model of spread used in implementation science, drawing on insights and a previous diagram in a review by Pierre Barker. Sources: Greenhalgh and Papoutsi, "Spreading and Scaling Up Innovation and Improvement; Barker, Reid, and Schall, "A Framework for Scaling Up Health Interventions: Lessons from Large-Scale Improvement Initiatives in Africa"

Finally, we would like to offer a few recommendations adapted from a systematic review of the implementation of e-health technologies[5] and mobile health tools.[6] There is gap between evidence and the practical aspects of integrating and implementing DTx into real-world clinical settings. Therefore, while evidence about implementing DTx are emerging, e-health technologies and mobile health tools, sharing

Important

A systematic effort to deploy an intervention *on a limited scale but across different settings* will help DTx organizations identify and deal with barriers that get in the way of the implementation effort and take advantage of facilitators that support it. The objective is ultimately to understand from an implementation standpoint not only the type of intervention that works to drive adoption but also answer the question on what works where and under what conditions.

Going Further with the NASSS Framework

To further your knowledge and understanding of implementation frameworks for new technologies, we recommend familiarizing yourself with the comprehensive nonadoption, abandonment, spread, scale-up, and sustainability (NASSS) framework. It can be used to inform the design of a new technology; identify solutions that have a limited chance of achieving sustained adoption; plan the implementation, scale-up, or rollout of a technology program; and learn from failures.[7]

technological and contextual similarities with DTx, can be used as a proxy to learn from on DTx implementation:

- Assess how each of the technology characteristics, such as its usability, adaptability to local contexts, and compatibility with existing systems, may affect the effectiveness of the implementation.
- Assess how the technology standards for interoperability, data security, and data privacy can improve acceptability and implementation (discussed in detail in chapter 6).
- Ensure there is sufficient financial and legislative support to assist implementation.
- Identify key stakeholders and knowledgeable champions with a track record of supporting and successfully advancing promising new health technologies, and include them early on in the design, planning, and implementation process.

- Provide reliable educational and training materials about the technology's features, benefits, and workflow integration scenarios aimed not only at primary users (i.e., physicians and patients) but at all individuals and entities involved in paying for and using the technology (i.e., employers, health plans, etc.).
- Support an overall cultural shift at the clinic/point-of-care that promotes the benefits of technology and innovation.
- Take a proactive, systematic, and global view of the implementation process. It must be considered at appropriate stages in the DTx development continuum given the multitude of segments involved in its successful execution. A well-planned implementation process ensures the state of readiness of end users and their organizations, as well as provides critical user feedback that can lead to dynamic procedural adjustments that can catalyze or potentially preclude adoption. For example, new roles supporting technology implementation may be required at the clinic (as well as within the DTx organization), with multidisciplinary teams combining digital and clinical expertise.

Conclusion

Testing, implementing, and ultimately scaling up DTx are not easy tasks. The implementation of DTx solutions does not conclude with a going-live announcement or with a press release, as we see too often. It should be considered a comprehensive process, not an event.

Following an IS approach and taking the implementation process through a sequence of activities (such as involving health care system managers early on) and appropriate support mechanisms will facilitate the adoption of interventions and empower the solution to work at its full potential in a specific context. DTx solutions, like any other innovation that aspires to be sustainably adopted over time, will need to adapt to their unique local environments dynamically. As a result, the DTx implementation strategy must be monitored and modulated, and the underlying technology evaluated, on an ongoing basis to ensure that intended goals are met, benefits are realized, and barriers to effective use are identified and addressed.

NOTES

1. NUHS is a group of Singapore health care institutions composed of several hospitals, national specialty centers, and polyclinics.

2. Mathews and Yadron, "Health Insurer Anthem Hit by Hackers."

3. Plsek, "Redesigning Health Care with Insights from the Science of Complex Adaptive Systems."

4. Implementation outcomes such as acceptability, adoption, costs, or penetration are indicators of implementation success but not of treatment effectiveness. They should therefore only be considered as "intermediate outcomes," which serve as necessary preconditions for attaining subsequent desired changes in patient's clinical outcomes.

5. Ross et al., "Factors that Influence the Implementation of e-Health."

6. Jacob, Sanchez-Vazquez, and Ivory, "Social, Organizational, and Technological Factors Impacting Clinicians' Adoption of Mobile Health Tools."

7. Greenhalgh et al., "Beyond Adoption."

CHAPTER 10

Supporting Adoption of DTx

This chapter was coauthored by Dr. Robyn Mildon, Founding Executive Director of the Centre for Evidence and Implementation with offices in Australia, Singapore, and the United Kingdom.

The reality is that many of the envisioned solutions in health care are not widely adopted or scalable (enough) to put into practice, and any proposed changes to current practices—like a new technology—has multiple barriers to overcome. Will things be different for DTx? Will this increasingly prevalent approach smoothly implement itself? Given its intended role in transforming the delivery and administration of medical care, this is unlikely. DTx organizations need to be proactive in their implementation efforts and take learnings from other technologies that are being implemented and adopted (or not) in health care. In this chapter, we provide two perspectives, those of health professionals and those of patients, for how DTx can achieve buy-in. The two often go hand in hand, in a virtuous cycle. We share here what we believe are the key considerations and factors—often beyond the technology itself—to enter that cycle to catalyze and sustain DTx adoption.

Achieving Clinical Adoption of DTx

Acceptance by health care professionals may be the single most important determinant of whether a new health technology or service succeeds.[1] Understanding the reasons for potential resistance to using and prescribing DTx and finding ways in which DTx organizations can support DTx acceptance and adoption among clinicians is, therefore, imperative.

One of the physicians interviewed by our team noted, "Doctors are early adopters of technology that works and that they understand." Physicians recognize the value of new drugs and medical device innovations, such as small pacemakers. With increased exposure to digital health platforms, doctors are also becoming more accepting of platforms into the patient care repertoire. According to a survey from the American Medical Association, the use and appreciation of information technology and digital health tools by physicians in general has seen a substantial increase between 2016 and 2019. This includes the category of remote monitoring and management for improved care solutions, to which DTx belongs.[2]

Having said that, health care startups often fail to understand physicians' perspectives, which gives rise to some of the unforeseen barriers to adopting DTx that the DTx designers discover down the road. For example, with the technology evolving so rapidly and algorithms-driven decision-making processes requiring more clarity, physicians may need substantial support in sufficiently assessing and, ultimately, trusting the technology. Additionally, digital health is often associated with increased data management demands that add more administrative burden to the clinicians' daily practice, potentially challenging or even discouraging adoption. Following is an overview of the key issues that should be anticipated and addressed proactively to engage and prepare physicians to embrace technology-enabled health care.

Identifying High-Priority Needs

Empowering physician buy-in for an emerging technology starts with demonstrated abilities to solve established challenges in their daily practice. For example, for British primary care physicians, one of the most common issues their patients present with, and for which there is currently no agreed-upon treatment, is insomnia.

> *Insomnia is common and debilitating, yet despite 10% prevalence there is no gold standard treatment in the UK that is readily available for prescription or referral in the NHS [National Health Service]. There is a massive treatment gap that physicians want to solve. At Big Health, we provided physicians with Sleepio, a DTx for insomnia, backed by 12 randomized controlled trials—the gold standard when it comes to scientific evidence. We also partnered with organizations to provide physicians with sleep and DTx education—how to assess for insomnia, which patients are indicated for our DTx solution, how to support patients, and when to follow up. The DTx has to be embedded into existing clinical pathways, rather than being introduced as an "app."* —Dr. Charlotte Lee, UK Director, Big Health, a DTx company that develops solutions for mental health.[3]

DTx implementation requires early interest from physicians. As you might expect, if your DTx solution offers to address physicians' top clinical priorities, you'll have a better chance of securing their time for a product demonstration and education sessions—key entry points for subsequent pathways toward integration into a clinical workflow. These sessions, also referred to as physician training and education, provide opportunities to continuously communicate the results of various studies and clinical trials regarding the safety and effectiveness of solutions that are already mature. It's the first step to gaining physician trust and avoiding physician bias.

It is also strongly advised to involve physicians as early as possible throughout the DTx development and implementation stages. This level of proactive engagement helps to ensure that DTx platforms address their needs while also helping them to gain a foundational understanding of the technology and how to use it effectively. These engagements will increase physicians' overall confidence in DTx and drive ownership, ultimately empowering physician adoption.

Anticipating Workflow Changes

Recent studies looking at how physicians divide their time daily found that for every hour dedicated to providing direct clinical care to patients, they spend up to three additional hours on administrative work.[4] How DTx technologies are incorporated into established clinical workflows is therefore critical to ensuring that they do not create additional burden for physicians. This is important as high patient loads result in physicians spending a substantial portion of their time looking at their screens and away from their patients, which can subsequently impact the patient-physician relationship.

And just as we are now discussing the changes that a DTx may introduce to existing workflows and communications, we also need to evaluate its compatibility with future workflows, future upgrades to the infrastructure that would support it, and future needs of the health care staff that would use and recommend it to their patients. DTx may disrupt existing patterns of team interaction in ways that can prove to be more complex than initially anticipated.[5] The adoption of DTx often involves multiple stakeholders, numerous decision-making processes, potentially novel routes for communication between care teams or between care teams and patients and caregivers, as well as a series of personal and organizational value judgements. From past experiences with introducing new technology into a clinical setting, we have observed that clinical and administrative staff are vital when it comes to integrating innovations into everyday clinic use. Consequently, patients are more likely to take advantage of, and benefit from, such interventions if clinical staff have been extensively involved with vetting and facilitating the onboarding process and if the intervention has been introduced by staff members who recognized its capacity for markedly improved patient outcomes over traditional approaches.[6]

Addressing DTx-Driven Changes in the Patient-Physician Relationship

In the 1980s and 1990s, artificial intelligence (AI) was perceived as a not-so-subtle threat represented by the *Terminator* and *Matrix* movie series. But in 2020 and beyond, instead of taking the form of a menacing robot or omnipresent authoritarian, AI is more likely to take on the form of recommended purchases on Amazon or targeted Facebook ads. Concerns about technology's impact on our everyday lives have evolved too, expanding from the influences it can wield in our digital and online environments to affecting how we engage in person-to-person interactions, especially in health care. And in the realm of health care, these fears can sometimes morph into worry that digitizing health care—whether by bringing in surgical robots or DTx—will replace both physicians and the human connection they forge with their patients. As a result of the workflow changes outlined in the previous section, it is necessary to consider how DTx may ultimately affect the patient-physician interaction in some way.

Patients' motivations for visiting a doctor usually encompass much more than a desire to receive a medical report about their health state and recommendations on how to continue to care for themselves. The compassion, empathy, and reassurance they expect, and often receive, from their physicians have been shown to have a substantial impact on both the individual's health outcomes and the health care system's own outcomes (including economic).[7] These benefits would be too precious to lose if a digitally powered health care system was perceived to somehow constrain such personal patient-doctor interactions. DTx solutions should be carefully incorporated into existing health care modalities so as not to disrupt any positive patient-doctor interactions that have already been established but instead aim to support and potentially even improve their quality (e.g., through increased accessibility), where possible.

In an ideal DTx-empowered clinical practice scenario, such technologies would serve to automatically generate information about disease evolution, assessment, and treatment plans, thereby freeing up time to discuss what really matters to a patient—their life and how the disease impacts it. By shifting most of the informational and educational workload from the physician and empowering the patient, DTx platforms can facilitate the provision of care beyond basic medical needs, and as such have the potential to improve human connections.

Addressing the Cost Issue

As mentioned, insomnia care may be a high-priority need for physicians, yet during our interviews with health care professionals, one physician, referring to the financing of DTx implementation and usage, promptly asked us, "Who will bear the cost?" It is a critical question for any DTx solutions, and the solution starts with demonstrating the intervention's cost-effectiveness. For example, a recent study looked at the cost-effectiveness of digitally administered cognitive behavioral treatment (CBT) for insomnia (Sleepio).[8] The study looked at both direct and indirect costs—including treatment expenses, insomnia-related health care expenses, and the costs of reduced productivity at the workplace. The quality-adjusted life years (QALYs), which is an established method of determining the value of health care treatments, was designated by this study as US$50,000. This work also compared different forms of intervention against digitally administered CBT (including pharmacologic intervention, group CBT, single patient CBT, and no treatment). The study demonstrated that digital CBT was the most cost-effective treatment, but it also had the highest positive net monetary benefit (NMB) relative to no insomnia treatment (i.e., $681.06 for each patient over a six-month period). More specifically, the NMB term served as a measure of the value of a treatment in a monetary context when there was an established threshold for a willingness to pay. In other words, a positive NMB shows that the cost of realizing the benefit is less than the maximum amount that a decision-maker (e.g., insurance company) would be willing to reimburse to achieve this benefit.

Beyond the cost-effectiveness aspects, would the DTx be covered under a specific benefit, whether pharmacy, medical, or even value-based contracting? Would the patient's insurance pay for it? Or would it be covered by patients out of pocket? The question of cost, who bears it, and the cost-effectiveness in the adoption of DTx is crucial. A systematic review of 221 studies looking at the factors influencing success and failure of e-health interventions found that cost was the most frequently reported contributing factor to failure.[9]

Although new technologies in general and DTx in particular are commonly portrayed as long-term cost-saving opportunities, their implementation and the learning curve they require for deployment often imply the opposite. Patients may still need to take their pills and continue to see their physicians as usual while both sides get comfortable enough with the technology for it to replace the conventional care pathway. This is due to the fact that some of the challenges that consistently bedevil health care include staff shortages and a generalized dearth of training, space, and equipment. Yet to fully integrate DTx into new clinical workflows, health care providers need to "go digital" by transitioning to appropriate infrastructures that drive digital services and developing other digital-centric capabilities.

In a nutshell, this is one of the few points on which all stakeholders in the DTx ecosystem will agree: DTx must be cost-effective and aligned with value-based medicine. DTx must therefore build a case for long-term savings while also addressing the upfront expenses of the technology induction period and the ongoing costs.

Supporting Patient Adoption of DTx
Having the Right Engagement Strategy

There is growing literature on how engaged patients are more likely to be proactive and empowered in their care, understand their condition, and ultimately adopt new healthy behaviors—a profoundly important and elusive outcome. The key finding from these studies is that higher incidence of patient engagement is associated with improved health outcomes.[10] It also positively impacts the patients' and clinicians' experiences and delivery of care. So what does an effective patient engagement strategy look like in the digital age?

Today, the patient-physician interaction is frequently the primary determinant of the patient experience. The personalization of this experience is often limited to adjustments to the treatment plan (e.g., changes to regimen, dose titration, etc.). A DTx, on the other hand, can provide a broad spectrum of new digital channels and, as a result, new digital delivery mechanisms to drive engagement with both providers and patients. For example, providers can potentially tap into digitally enabled channels to sustainably communicate and engage with patients to disseminate content or track symptoms. DTx developers can also collect real-time patient information (e.g., self-reported outcomes, patient feedback systems, emotion tracking, etc.) to engage patients proactively and/or in a more timely and personalized manner, leveraging a wide range of data and information.

These new digital touchpoints and interactions across channels provide new engagement strategies. Personalized nudges, online support groups, connected caregivers and families, bite-sized e-learning, digitally shared decision-making interventions, and potential instant gratification through gamification elements are just a few emerging patient engagement strategies, each with a different level of maturity and evidence. These resources serve as potential catalysts toward achieving truly personalized patient treatment as well as engagement experiences. This can, in turn, empower patients, drive sustained use of the DTx, and ultimately achieve better treatment outcomes compared to conventional strategies. This is echoed by recent insights shared in our contributor interviews following a COVID-19 use case. "We used to send daily reminders to COVID-19 patients for symptoms reporting, but we realized after some time that most patients had formed habits and we really only needed to send them reminders when they forgot to report their readings," said Dorothea Koh, founder and CEO of BotMD, which powers Singapore's National University Health System virtual wards program to care for COVID-19 patients remotely.[11]

One relevant approach to patient engagement for DTx is an omnichannel approach that fully leverages these new touchpoints. It is defined as a multichannel patient engagement strategy that will collect and aggregate all clinical and nonclinical data and information generated by these new touchpoints and interactions. This integration of systems, channels, and information creates a single view of the patient and for the patient. It provides unique insights into their treatments, also revealing a full picture of a patient's health profile beyond only clinical aspects. It also offers the possibility to take into consideration the range of personal, social, economic, and environmental factors influencing a patient's health. For example, emotions have been shown to alter judgment and decision-making.[12] So how can DTx account for emotional ups and downs that patients experience to personalize the engagement experience? Since there isn't a one-size-fits-all patient engagement strategy, and offering patients individualized content and intervention is essential for building stronger engagement, and probably better outcomes, an omnichannel approach may serve as a suitable solution.

The omnichannel approach has been mastered by retail and e-commerce players, offering a seamless shopping experience both online and in-store. Integration across several touchpoints (i.e., physical stores, websites, product pages, apps, mobile ads, and other means) is critical for generating data, traffic, and, eventually, sales. For DTx, there are two main goals, closely interconnected. The first goal is to create a seamless and personalized experience that meets patients where they are—the possibility to address issues that matter to them and respond to their preferences, needs, and values. The second goal is to empower patients in their own care, increase adherence to a therapy, and encourage behavior change, with the ultimate goal of improving outcomes.

We should emphasize that incorporating patient engagement strategies should not be considered only when patients are first prescribed a DTx. In fact, these strategies should be addressed from the very beginning of the solution's design phase. It's a multistage process from pre- to post-intervention (i.e., activation, sustained use, and weaning off the DTx when the treatment is finished). A robust and effective DTx patient engagement strategy should also be developed with a user-centric approach. For example, the Patient Centered Outcomes Research Institute created a "patient co-investigator" role for their studies. Patients are more than study participants. In fact, they are vital stakeholders empowering the research studies that could include the design of a new digital health intervention that could impact their own health journeys.[13] As such, effective patient engagement approaches can help DTx developers comprehend factors and design elements to drive sustained use of the solution and ultimately support positive user experiences and outcomes.

Strengthening Relationships

In a health care context, DTx solutions should strengthen relationships—the relationship between a patient and physician and the relationship between the patients and their own health. These relationships play a vital role in driving and sustaining DTx adoption, and reinforcing these relationships involves understanding the emotional aspects that underlie the decisions patients make in consultation with their doctors and on their own. For example, patients signing up for a digital health program through a physician referral, an employee assistance program, and an app store may have different expectations and motivations. As Dr. Lee shared with us, "Patients first need to acknowledge that they have a concern or a problem before deciding that they need to see a physician. When this is acted upon, their motivation to accept the recommended solution by their physician—be it a drug, an app, or a referral to a different service—is high. The two elements, trust and authority, are critical in this patient-physician relationship. The challenge for DTx, such as Big Health, is how to take this motivation and transform it into something scalable and accessible."

Trust is central to DTx uptake, as can be observed when would-be users hesitate to embrace a technology if they feel it is "faceless" or lacking a "human touch." Fortunately, this trust can be fostered by a third party; evidence shows that seeing a trusted person—a friend, family member, or a highly visible public figure—already using the DTx would often lead to interest in and engagement with the program. For this reason, Big Health decided to involve "link workers"—nonclinical social care practitioners embedded in primary care practices—to engage with and support patients who have been prescribed their apps. According to Dr. Lee, the retention rate for Sleepio, the company's DTx for poor sleep, rose substantially in Scotland with that model.

Trust in DTx solutions can also be engendered through connecting with other users of the same technology. Some companies are offering patients the opportunity to be part of a peer community as a built-in functionality of their platform and user interface. This approach has been found to be an effective method of improving engagement and achieving higher adherence rates compared with unsupported interventions.[14]

As a case in point, in one study looking at the effectiveness of virtual reality–based rehabilitative stroke therapy, researchers found that stroke patients training in the multiuser version of the system, which provided the ability to connect with others online, showed greater adoption compared to the same patients training in the single-user mode. Specifically, patients spent up to 22% more time when using the multiuser version.[15] In another study, 30% of tobacco users who enrolled in a digital program that worked with a health coach managed to quit for good, compared to the 20% who did so after engaging only with digital tools.[16]

Many DTx today, in our opinion, lack an essential hook as part of their offering—the ability for users to connect with someone like them, someone who could empathize with their health care journey because they have the same health condition or lived experience with a disease. PatientsLikeMe, an online community where patients exchange thoughts and advice for managing a variety of diseases with others, embodies the concept well. However, this community differs from a DTx. Peer support, including online peer support communities, is gaining popularity as a means of supplementing the self-management of chronic health conditions. It can be a valuable source of information and a safe haven for patients, frequently extending beyond medical care. As proof of their effectiveness emerges, expect DTx to embrace such features.

Celebrating Success with Short-Term Wins

Remember Fabien, his daily struggles to manage his type 1 diabetes, and his rollercoaster of emotions? His physician advised him that his main objective was to manage his blood sugar levels—not the most exciting or engaging task from Fabien's perspective. Frequent reminders from the physician and from his family about the risk of suffering kidney failure or a foot amputation if he fails to manage his condition well was not helping his morale, either. To stay motivated, he needed concrete, trackable, and achievable short- and long-term objectives. As he noted during our interview, "What if I want to climb Mount Everest? What if this is my objective and not managing diabetes or getting my blood sugar under control? Tell me what I need to do, the steps required so that I can ultimately be successful at climbing Mount Everest."

Indeed, Fabien's definition of success, which is to climb Mount Everest, will almost certainly not coincide with his physician's definition of success, which is to improve his health outcomes, clinically speaking. Success from the perspective of a physician caring for a diabetes patient is primarily based on lowering the patient's glycemic variability, while from the perspective of the patient, success is based on managing their condition with as little effort as possible so that they can accomplish other personal or professional goals that are meaningful to them while having a minimal effect on their daily routines (figure 10.1).

As definitions of successful disease management differ depending on who we ask, we invite DTx designers to consider both patient and physician perspectives on how a DTx solution could benefit each party and help them achieve their respective goals and objectives. In addition to taking the long view, DTx designers also need to ensure their

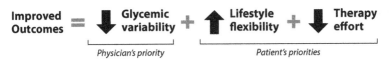

FIGURE 10.1. Improved outcomes for a diabetes patient is a combination of both physician priorities and patient priorities. Source: From the authors

technology is delivering enough short-term wins—symbolically celebrating hitting predetermined milestones along the way—in order to keep users involved. These acknowledgments could be designed to take place right when the DTx is introduced to the patient for the first time, within the first few weeks of them using the therapy, or periodically during the course of treatment. The idea is to provide psychological reinforcement for any positive changes in behavior, symptoms, or clinical outcomes that the DTx is able to accurately capture and track longitudinally.

Nudge Me Right!

Human nature does not always produce the rational decision-makers we may hope to be. When it comes to managing even our own health, we don't always have the willpower to stay the course on a treatment regimen, exercise, or diet plan. Rigorous cost-benefit analyses and trade-offs between immediate gratification and future health outcomes often go out the window when we face the option of doing something that puts a physical or psychological burden on us, as one might find with trying to adhere to a workout plan or a demanding daily therapy. Luckily, these natural biases in the decision-making process can be turned into an advantage by encouraging health-enhancing behaviors through the use of "nudges."

The word *nudge* was popularized when the Cameron government introduced the Behavioural Insights Team in the UK—also known as the Nudge Unit—to investigate how desirable behavior could be encouraged. In a nutshell, nudging attempts to subtly lead people toward making the right decision. It can be used to encourage behaviors that are beneficial to one's health compared to a common default behavior that could be construed as a bad habit. For example, instead of outright banning junk-food advertising, nudging can change the order in which options are presented, with healthier options listed first to subconsciously steer consumers' attention to healthier choices.

The same principle can be applied in the context of making health-related decisions. How can patients' environments be tweaked so as to help them make healthier choices? For example, changing a choice architecture default by requiring people to opt out of organ donation rather than opt in may lead to more organ donations and more lives saved.[17] In the same vein, Penn Medicine in 2014 switched its electronic health record system's default from brand-name drugs to their generic equivalents. This immediately increased generic prescribing rates from 75% to 98%, leading to a $32 million savings to both patients and the health system within two and a half years.[18] Common behavior mechanisms used to nudge patients are listed in table 10.1.

Closer to DTx, Livongo—which offers chronic disease management programs, including for diabetes by combining connected devices, data sharing, and coaching—is a good example of a digital health technology built on the principle of nudging. By the end of 2019, the company had delivered 2 million "Health Nudges," which they defined in their preliminary prospectus with the US Securities and Exchange Commission as "small, readily accessible interventions, which can include hundreds of different behavior or lifestyle adjustments that can alter clinical outcomes for people with a chronic condition, such as diet advice, medication information, or suggestions for increases in physical activity. People simply want to live their lives, not be constantly reminded that they are living with a condition."[19]

Livongo's health nudges work by detecting a behaviorally modifiable issue that could lead to worse health outcomes if left unaddressed and sending out a suggestion for corrective action. For example, when the system identifies a user that has not been checking their blood glucose in the mornings, a nudge is sent to encourage them to do so before breakfast in order to better understand overnight patterns.

Table 10.1. Behavior mechanisms to nudge patient

Changing defaults	Individuals prefer sticking to existing or standard behaviors rather than doing something different or involving an effortful choice.
	Example: Opt-in vs. opt-out strategies for organ donation.
Hyperbolic discounting	Individuals prefer short-term rewards, do not like uncertainty and will try to reduce it whenever possible, and tend to undervalue less concrete future rewards.
	Example: Rewarding an increase in steps, logging blood glucose, and light exercise vs. an HbA1c reduction after three months.
Loss and risk aversion	Individuals are reluctant to take risks and accept potential losses, unless this can be compensated by potential important rewards. In other words, they do not mind not having something, but they do mind losing something.
	Example: Whenever attempting to change patient behaviors, health care professionals need to be able to explain the benefits and gains to their patients, and contrast it with the losses, so that these can be tangibly assessed.
Framing	Decision-making is perceived as easier when a few options are available, but at the same time, having too many options can be counterproductive.
	Example: Choices should always be framed in ways that help patients and staff understand what their preferences are.
Reciprocity	Individuals strive to reciprocate commitments. They are more likely to change their behaviors if they feel that they owe someone else something.
	Example: Studies that applied this principle to health care issues found that organ donations could be increased significantly after a campaign containing the message "If you needed an organ transplant would you have one?"
Social norms and feedback (or peer pressure influence)	Individuals tend to base their behaviors on what they perceive others are doing, comparing themselves and what they think they are expected to do in order to conform to the norm. Feedback on how individual performance evolves over time can help while also improving behaviors.
	Example: Instead of saying "Please arrive on time," state that "80% of patients in this clinic arrive on time for their appointments." Communicating the percentage of patients who arrive on time for their appointment has been showed to decrease no-shows by as much as 30%.

Source: Voyer, "'Nudging' Behaviours in Healthcare."

These interventions are provided through the member's preferred communication channel (e.g., a blood glucose meter, a mobile app, the web, or email) and are based on an analysis of patient-generated information collected over time, such as self-reported data and data generated from wearables and sensors. The analysis consists of scanning for patterns that help to select the type of nudge that would be most effective in a particular context and for a particular individual. Livongo noted that its health nudges lead patients to make smarter health choices and drive behavior changes: "Over 40% of our members who received a Health Nudge changed their behavior in response to a suggestion that they complete a blood glucose check before breakfast."[20]

Penn Medicine and Livongo's use of nudges demonstrate how strategies and tools borrowed from the field of psychology can be leveraged to influence patient behavior. However, nudging is just a tool that is part of the solution to better disease management, but not *the* solution. A multifaceted approach is necessary to create an engaging technology that steers patients to make healthier decisions, and motivates physicians to endorse and prescribe new DTx solutions.

Conclusion

As more data emerge on user engagement with DTx, it is critical for innovators to take these into account and respond adaptively by removing, adding, or improving upon features that lead to better motivation, sustained use, and clinical outcomes. To achieve this, it is important to involve physicians and patients as early as possible, where appropriate, in the development and deployment of DTx. This cocreation approach to explore existing problems and potential solutions holistically can substantially improve the likelihood of a DTx platform being adopted. Put simply, people support what they have helped create.

NOTES

1. Greenhalgh et al., "Beyond Adoption."
2. Miliard, "AMA Sees Surge in Health IT Adoption, 'Rise of the Digital-Native Physician.'"
3. From an in interview with the authors, October 26, 2021.
4. Wenger et al., "Allocation of Internal Medicine Resident Time in a Swiss Hospital"; Sinsky et al., "Allocation of Physician Time in Ambulatory Practice."
5. Greenhalgh et al., "Beyond Adoption."
6. Aref-Adib et al., "Factors Affecting Implementation of Digital Health Interventions for People with Psychosis or Bipolar Disorder, and Their Family and Friends."
7. Trzeciak and Mazzarelli, *Compassionomics: The Revolutionary Scientific Evidence that Caring Makes a Difference*; Derksen, Bensing, and Lagro-Janssen, "Effectiveness of Empathy in General Practice."

8. Darden et al., "Cost-Effectiveness of Digital Cognitive Behavioral Therapy (*Sleepio*) for Insomnia."

9. Granja, Janssen, and Johansen, "Factors Determining the Success and Failure of eHealth Interventions."

10. Greene et al., "When Patient Activation Levels Change, Health Outcomes and Costs Change, Too"; Krist et al., "Engaging Patients in Decision-Making and Behavior Change to Promote Prevention"; Bombard et al., "Engaging Patients to Improve Quality of Care."

11. From an interview with the authors, May 19, 2022.

12. Lerner et al., "Emotion and Decision Making."

13. Robbins, Tufte, and Hsu, "Learning to 'Swim' with the Experts."

14. Aref-Adib et al., "Factors Affecting Implementation of Digital Health Interventions for People with Psychosis or Bipolar Disorder, and Their Family and Friends."

15. Thielbar et al., "Home-Based Upper Extremity Stroke Therapy Using a Multiuser Virtual Reality Environment."

16. "VP Live," Virgin Pulse.

17. Davidai, Gilovich, and Ross, "The Meaning of Default Options for Potential Organ Donors."

18. Levins, "Report from the First National 'Nudge Units in Health Care' Symposium."

19. Livongo Health, "United States Securities and Exchange Commission Form S-1 Registration Statement," 3.

20. Livongo Health, "United States Securities and Exchange Commission Form S-1 Registration Statement," 131.

PART IV

PATHS TO COMMERCIALIZATION

This part was coauthored with Christopher Hardesty. Hardesty is a partner at Pureland Venture in Singapore who specializes in building early-stage medical innovations for scale-up in Asia and beyond. He has lived and worked in more than 50 countries to design public-private health system financial schemes, including for the creation of pathways for the adoption of medical innovations.

Pre-COVID-19, we knew a fundamentally new approach was required to transform our health care systems and respond to the rise in chronic and mental health diseases and their consequences. Regulators, payers, and prescribers were starting to learn about DTx as a valid therapy alternative or complement for the treatment of a variety of illnesses.

With the recent adoption of digital health and models for delivering health care remotely, we have seen a variety of new commercialization strategies being undertaken by early-stage and established manufacturers of DTx. Since the COVID-19 emergence, the US Food and Drug Administration (FDA) has exempted many regulatory requirements for DTx treating psychiatric disorders, such as the need to file a 510(k) premarket notice. Within a week, Akili Interactive made its DTx for ADHD available to qualified families at no cost and without the need for a doctor's prescription. Simultaneously, Corey McCann, CEO of Pear Therapeutics, stated that teleprescribing for its therapies had "gone through the roof." The pandemic did, in fact, generate new collaboration possibilities and care models as individuals sought care in places other than hospitals, such as patients' homes and communities. In summary, the broader health care ecosystem is appreciating more and more the potential of DTx. Is a health care revolution underway?

In 2019, the global DTx market was valued at $2.69 billion.[1] In 2020 alone, several DTx solutions achieved meaningful early scale, including new rounds of funding with $1.2 billion across 52 deals in 2019,[2] including mergers, partnerships, and high-profile product launches in the United States, European Union, and Asia. According to MedRhythms, the DTx industry went from having about 13 new products a year between 2012 and 2015, to 44 a year between 2016 and 2019, to 80 in 2020 alone.[3] There was also a significant uptake of DTx for neuropsychiatric indications from 2012 to 2020 (figure Part IV-1).

The global DTx market is expected to reach $11.82 billion by 2027, growing at a compound annual growth rate of 20.3% during the 2020–2027 period.[4] DTx are certainly gaining traction, but what would it take for DTx to achieve meaningful scale and play a pivotal role in the transformation of our health systems?

Despite the notable successes of a few DTx technologies in terms of conceptualization, regulatory clearance, and early adoption, all too often achieving scalable commercial success remains a hard-to-reach reality. Perhaps the best known example of the elusive nature of success for DTx organizations is Proteus, the "smart pill" startup that

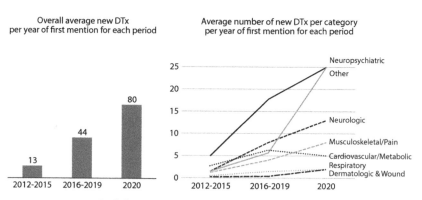

FIGURE PART IV.1. Proliferation of DTx products. Source: McCarthy, "Looking Back & Ahead at the Digital Therapeutics Industry"

was once considered a unicorn because of its US$1.5 billion valuation but then filed for bankruptcy in 2020.[5] For nearly two decades, Proteus had planned to revolutionize medication adherence with its ingestible sensor—a tiny microchip the size of a grain of sand that could be planted into any drug and send signals to a smartphone app and a digital portal to inform if the pill was swallowed or not. But as it sought to cross the chasm between being a new, little-known exploratory product and becoming a widely adopted recognized solution, the organization suffered from two common blind spots:

1. *Lack of full channel understanding.* In the case of Proteus, the eagerness to quickly go to market led the company to prematurely strike a deal with the Japanese multinational company Otsuka Pharmaceutical. The objective of the deal was to become a leader in the emerging category of "digital medicines" by pairing up with Otsuka's popular antipsychotic drug Abilify (aripiprazole), approved for treating various neurological conditions in adults. There were many challenges with this drug–device pairing, such as the fact that people with schizophrenia, for whom Abilify is frequently prescribed, tend to fear being controlled or monitored, which in a way is what Proteus's DTx was designed to do. Even if the partnership made technological sense, the company lacked a comprehensive understanding of motivations and potential objections of the sensor-equipped drug's primary users, influencers, and purchasers, including the various partners who would help distribute and commercialize the solution (the channel partners).[6]

2. *Value exchange that is not fit for the purpose.* Any DTx innovator seeking to commercialize their invention must eventually grapple with the pricing question. Exacerbating the lack of channel understandings for Proteus—referring to its distribution system—was the fact that Abilify cost roughly 80 times more than cheaper drug alternatives. Therefore, the task for Proteus to demonstrate equivalent if not better health outcomes

and economic returns became essentially insurmountable. As the FDA recognized in the wake of the drug's commercial failure, "Regulatory approval for this first-ever digital drug was based on weak evidence, with no evidence of better adherence with the digital version of aripiprazole compared with the non-digital version. Both the scientific literature and news reports conveyed an unsupported impression of benefit."[7]

Being on the front line of health care innovation is never easy, as the Proteus case demonstrates. Rather than being disheartened, let us seek to learn from such prior experiences in order to improve the scalable success rate of what is an unavoidable positive trend toward DTx innovation in the health care industry. In chapter 11, we focus on channel partnerships as one of the most effective paths to commercialization and discuss channel partnership strategies by types, mechanisms for engagement, and best practices therein. The goal of channel partnerships is to optimize a DTx product's distribution and commercialization strategy, and we provide suggestions on how to maintain momentum and ramp up your commercialization journey as you hit adoption milestones along the way. In chapter 12, we focus on the payers. We explore for the concept of value, especially the economic value of DTx, and how it might be demonstrated to private and public payers. As value lies in the eye of the beholder and is market-specific, it is critical to understand how such value is defined from various payers' perspectives, and therefore the evidence that will be required to convince potential payers of the necessity of a DTx solution.

NOTES

1. Precedence Research, "Digital Therapeutics Market Size to Hit US$ 11.82 Bn by 2027."

2. Bridge Point Capital, "Advancement of Digital Therapeutics Leads to a Huge Market with Enormous Potential."

3. McCarthy, "Looking Back & Ahead at the Digital Therapeutics Industry."

4. Precedence Research, "Digital Therapeutics Market Size to Hit US$ 11.82 Bn by 2027."

5. Farr, "Proteus Digital Health, Once Valued at $1.5 Billion, Files for Chapter 11 Bankruptcy."

6. Muoio, "Proteus Parts Ways with Otsuka as It Pivots toward Oncology, Infectious Disease Treatment Adherence."

7. Cosgrove et al., "Digital Aripiprazole or Digital Evergreening?"

Channel Partnerships

The Ultimate Commercialization Strategy

After considering how DTx adoption might be predicted and assisted in the previous chapter, it is time to consider the significance of DTx partnerships in the commercialization of the solution. The go-to-market models may be quite particular to your therapeutic area and intervention, but they may also differ from market to market.

To date, three business models have emerged as dominant in the digital health and digital wellness space: business-to-consumer (B2C), business-to-business (B2B), and business-to-business-to-consumer (B2B2C). B2C is a model of choice for technologies that do not require regulatory clearance, are not prescription-based, and can be purchased "over the digital counter" of an app store by the end users. B2B and B2B2C are models of choice for technologies that undergo higher level of scrutiny and that have a differential approach to reimbursement. Those models are nonexclusive and both require a structured approach to planning, organizing, and executing the business strategy.

We have seen DTx innovators opting for not one channel but a multichannel distribution approach and therefore pursuing more than one business model, either concurrently or sequentially. This approach allows one to reach a range of users and diversify revenue streams, which is of particular importance for companies that have just brought a product to market. For example:

- **AEvice Health**, the previously mentioned Singapore-based remote-monitoring company operating in the field of respiratory illness, is pursuing the B2C route so as to gain experience and build a foundational dataset while planning for a regulated medical solution that will use distribution partners for scale-up support (B2B2C).
- **DarioHealth**, a DTx solution for chronic conditions, after gaining momentum in B2C models and showing the required clinical results at scale, transitioned to a B2B2C strategy, targeting employers, health plans (i.e., any program that helps patients pay for medical expenses, whether through privately purchased insurance, social insurance, or a social welfare program funded by the government), and providers.
- **Glooko**, a US-based software-as-a-service solution for diabetes management, launched both an FDA-cleared insulin dosing system paired with a mobile app for consumers (B2C) and a "kiosk"-style offering for in-clinic health care professionals that provide care for diabetes patients (B2B2C).

As you can see, the B2C model is a common way of introducing the company and the product to the market. However, while some level of direct selling may still be feasible at scale, true scalability across geographies, customer bases, and payment archetypes typically requires strategic partnerships with third parties. The good news is that identifying such entities may be easier now than it was before the pandemic. In the post-COVID-19 era, one often gets the impression that "every" business is pivoting into the health care industry, and whether that is justified or not, the positive artifact is that the universe of potential channel partners for DTx innovation is growing wider (table 11.1).

Each of these potential partners brings different assets, capabilities, and expertise. While some may be more suited to assist a DTx organ-

Table 11.1. Potential channel partners for large-scale DTx distribution and commercialization

Near-term mature commercial partners	• Life sciences organizations: mainly pharmaceutical and medical device companies and their distributors • Employers: typically, medium- to large-size private companies providing health insurance to their employees • Insurers: mostly private health and life insurers
Medium-term emerging commercial partners	• TeleX organizations: including telehealth, telemedicine, and telecare organizations
Longer-term emerging commercial partners (subject to country specificities and readiness)	• Telcos: large telecommunications firms investing heavily in health care • Big Tech: large technological companies seeking expansion to the area of health care

ization's journey toward broad reimbursement coverage, others present an alternative pathway to business model optimization and scalability. Still, regardless of their orientation, it is necessary to keep in mind that not all partnerships lead to the same revenue generation, as some revenue models are still being determined, and therefore carry an inherently higher risk.

Ultimately, a DTx organization must do its due diligence to determine whether partnering with a particular channel partner is a good strategic fit relative to its planned commercialization journey. To help frame how each partnership category should be evaluated, we cover their distinguishing characteristics, advantages, and disadvantages in greater detail next.

Life Sciences Organizations: The Natural Choice
Pharmaceutical Companies

The pharmaceutical industry is being disrupted. Pricing pressures, patent expiries, desire for greater patient and clinician engagement, and new forms of competition are forcing the industry to reevaluate its traditional commercialization models. The blockbuster model, in which hopes hinged on the extraordinary commercial success of a few

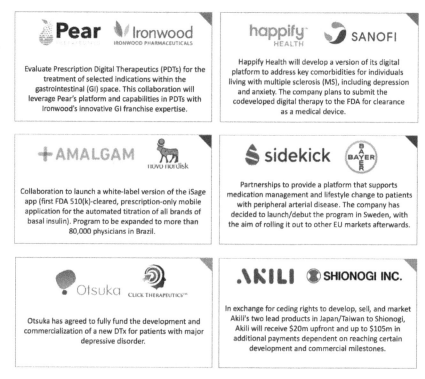

FIGURE 11.1. Examples of pharma–DTx partnerships for DTx development (*top row*), DTx commercialization (*middle row*), and DTx development plus commercialization (*bottom row*). Source: From the authors

billion-dollar-selling drugs, is slowly being challenged by real-world, data-driven, digitally supported therapeutic approaches like those embodied by DTx startups.

Having seen the writing on the wall, pharma companies are increasingly positioning themselves as a natural partner for DTx organizations throughout the clinical development, regulatory, and reimbursement pathways (figure 11.1). Granted, the go-to-market journey of a DTx product is very similar to that of a drug asset in terms of development, approval, commercialization, prescribing, and payment, so this type of partnership is the closest there is to a perfect match.

Pharma companies naturally see DTx partnerships as a win-win strategy, particularly when there is a close match between a drug and a software platform (a combination known in the industry vernacular as "drug-plus," whose aim is to improve clinical value by enhancing the drug's efficacy). One reason for that is such partnerships enable pharma organizations to differentiate themselves from competitors. In that frame of thinking, despite the eventual dissolution of the Proteus-Otsuka "marriage," the intentions that led to it were right—Abilify, which accounts for one quarter of Otsuka's total sales, lost its patent in 2015 and required an upgraded, differentiated approach to retain customers.[1]

Pharma industry players also need differentiation when it comes to engaging clinicians and key opinion leaders. Drug-plus programs or DTx that are positioned as a value-added service to existing therapies can be an interesting avenue to differentiation, on the condition that they can demonstrate superior value compared to conventional therapy alone. When looked at this way, DTx represents for pharma mainly some form of a companion platform rather than a new business stream. Hence, this type of pharma–DTx partnerships can take the form of copromotion or distribution arrangements instead of full-scale acquisitions. Much like in dating, the goal for both partners is to find an optimal strategic fit rather than base the union solely around financials.

Beyond differentiation, an ability to offer drug-plus programs fits into an evolving landscape of a health care solution offering. As the industry expands its focus from the clinical effectiveness of products, considered in isolation, to how those products fit into the broader chain of value-based care, engagement with patients and physicians plays a critical part. When done right, it can lead to better treatment adherence and, therefore, better health outcomes, effectively increasing a therapy's effectiveness. And engagement is becoming increasingly virtualized. Companion platforms provide an opportunity to increase patient engagement (remember our earlier discussion of nudges and behavioral change?), which in turn can have a direct positive revenue impact, since improved adherence tends to lead not only to better clinical outcomes, but also to higher sales. Through carefully structured data-sharing agreements, pharma companies may also gain the ability to obtain new data and insights about the clinical impact of their therapies across the care pathway; this is made possible by the data collection mechanisms embedded by design in DTx technologies. These real-word data, mediated through patient engagement and convertible into real-world evidence, have clinical as well as commercial value.

It is for all of these reasons that pharma players are often keen to acquire or partner with DTx startups from early development through to clinical validation and launch. There is a caveat, however. The revenue models for both—meaning the economic benefits for both players, DTx and the pharma—are yet to be demonstrated.

Medical Devices Companies

Like traditional pharma organizations, medical device companies (medtech) are similarly pressured into innovating their business models and their offerings. The Asia Pacific Medical Technology Association (APACMed), which brands itself as "the voice of MedTech in Asia," has seen several of its corporate members make significant investments in the DTx area. The association points to ResMed's acquisition of Propeller Health, which aims to pair ResMed's cloud-connectable medical devices for the treatment of sleep apnea and chronic obstructive pulmonary disease (COPD) with Propeller's DTx solutions for people living with COPD and asthma, as an example. Another collaboration, between Abbott and Sanofi, aims to simplify how people with diabetes manage their condition with smart pens, insulin titration apps, and cloud software.[2]

As medical device organizations are showing growing interest in partnering with DTx companies, in a parallel move a number of DTx and aspiring DTx companies have also joined the ranks of APACMed. Naluri and Wellthy Therapeutics, which provide clinically validated behavioral interventions for chronic disease management, are two of those early movers. While medtech and DTx have technological commonalities, both industries confront comparable obstacles in commercializing their "Software as a Medical Device" solutions.

Aside from the shift of medtech business models, medical devices are simply at the forefront of the digital revolution, with DTx being seen as attractive opportunities for more "connected" devices and toward better clinical outcomes. Many medtech companies position themselves as an attractive partner to DTx organizations that needs to be won over into the partnership. DTx entrepreneurs would be wise to develop their value proposition around how their solution provides value to the potential medtech partner. This is especially pertinent in the area of care pathways in which connected medical devices can play a role in patient monitoring and treatment adherence.

Delivering Value through Traditional Distribution Services

Finally, we must consider the life sciences organizations' distribution partners, including pharmacies, but also pharmaceutical distributors, such as McKesson, Zuellig Pharma, DKSH, and Takeda just to name a few. Squeezed between advanced, expensive therapies marketed by pharmaceutical companies and heightened pricing pressures by the payer and provider community, distributors must thread the needle of arriving at acceptable market prices while grappling with a complex, evolving supply chain of new health care solutions. Seeking to create value in such a dynamic marketplace, these distributors—traditionally seen as mere "box-pushers"—have been reinventing themselves from pure drug and medtech purveyors into integrated health care services groups. Some now offer full-suite health care services companies that include logistics, clinical trials, marketing, sales, insurance, and even digital and disease management solutions.

Zuellig Pharma, for example, is one of Asia's largest distributors of pharmaceutical products, serving over 350,000 medical facilities across 13 markets. Zuellig's transformation included a US$50 million investment in a Singapore-based innovation center in 2017 to develop data, digital, and disease management solutions that will assist doctors in developing more effective treatment plans, patients in managing chronic conditions, and payers in managing health care costs. In

2019, they also acquired the health tech firm Klinify, which provides a cloud-based digital medical assistant that assists over 800 Malaysian doctors in managing their clinics. The company stated that their objective is to leverage digital channels to supplement their existing companies and connect the health care ecosystem.[3] Whether through its own in-house development or through a variety of partnership deals, Zuellig, in addition to the reach and scale strategy, is building relevant and complementary capabilities to DTx solutions.

Final Thoughts on Life Sciences Organizations

Life science organizations have the infrastructure, market intelligence and expertise, dedicated salesforce, established relationships with key opinion leaders, payer contracting know-how, and evolving distribution systems that DTx ventures need to achieve scalability and widespread adoption. As such, they are ideally positioned as a natural channel partner for digital health innovators. Yet, despite the numerous benefits such partnerships may bring to DTx entrepreneurs, they also harbor risks.

Too many such cases as the previously discussed Proteus–Otsuka partnership, show how pharma–DTx collaborations may ultimately fail to achieve expectations if they originate from overexcitement and are not supported by a solid market research effort and business strategy. Pharma companies are themselves constantly evolving under the aforementioned pressures, so sometimes the existing salesforce incentives and key performance indicators, such as those aligned to the "blockbuster drug" mentality, are diverting leaders' attention away from championing the development of alternative approaches to selling a digital solution. Lack of firm commitment to resources, aggressive timelines, limited budget, and cross-marketing can also stifle potentially promising collaborations with DTx stakeholders.

On the other hand, DTx organizations' contributions to the pharma industry's financial performance is yet to be firmly demonstrated. The reason is that DTx products are not yet considered a turnkey solution that can be easily implemented into established business processes nor easily monetized over the next decade. Instead, their successful integration and commercialization requires iterative development and evidence generation.

Nevertheless, we remain optimistic about pharma, medtech players, and their associated distribution channels to serve as key commercial partners for DTx innovators. Partnerships between DTx and life sciences organizations must become entrenched and long-term, not just a step to get to the next round of funding. For this reason,

---

Pharma: A Partnership Example

Akili Interactive Labs, a DTx company that provides a prescription-based digital treatment for ADHD using a gamification approach, is an example of a company that concurrently pursues B2C and B2B2C distribution channels, depending on the market.

In 2019, to optimize their expansion to Asia, Akili announced a strategic partnership with Shionogi, a Japanese multinational pharmaceutical company specializing in treatments for pain and central nervous system disorders, to develop and commercialize DTx for the Japanese and Taiwanese markets.

Akili reiterated their desire to build a direct-to-consumer distribution model, with the announcement of a new Global Access Platform—a research and development as well as commercial platform—for all global product development activities. The platform also serves as an independent prescription and patient support system for DTx. Akili retained control of the core intellectual property platform that supports the commercialization of the DTx, as well as maintained stewardship of the data collected, in line with privacy standards. On the other hand, Shionogi is responsible for regulatory filings and has exclusive rights to the clinical development, sales, and marketing of the first two Akili DTx for ADHD and autism spectrum disorder in Japan and Taiwan.[4]

In short, the partnership sought to leverage each company's area of expertise in terms of building a new class of treatment for patients while ensuring a sound commercial model. This partnership for Akili probably demonstrates the necessity to have a multipronged approach, market by market, for the distribution and commercialization strategy of DTx.

DTx innovators are advised to choose their commercial and distribution partners wisely, and to retain strong cultures of innovation.

Employers: The Need for Speed?

In the countries that comprise the Organisation for Economic Co-operation and Development, approximately 65% of the working-age labor force are employed.[5] In the context of our discussion, this suggests that employers are a critical conduit for addressing the majority of working people's health and therapy needs. Employers, particularly in the United States and Asia, are increasingly expected to serve as health care enablers, mainly in the form of sponsoring health insurance, but also by providing prevention, wellness, and disease management solutions. In addition to footing the bill for many direct costs for health care and lost wages, respectively, employers and employees are collectively confronted with challenges associated with medical leave that can range from temporary to prolonged disability. Depression, for example, is estimated to cause 200 million lost workdays each year in the United States at a cost to employers of up to $44 billion.[6]

Employers benefit from a healthy, motivated workforce, both directly (e.g., lower insurance premiums) and indirectly (e.g., higher productivity). To further cultivate this work environment, employers started offering more general wellness platforms and lifestyle solutions to drive employee engagement and increase their general health literacy toward health screenings and preventive health. For example, while the impact of COVID-19 on patient health from an infectious disease standpoint was a huge challenge in itself, the pandemic's role as a driver of mental health challenges may not be anywhere close to being fully realized. With the emergence of the pandemic, DTx solutions for mental health have gained substantial visibility with the community at large, but also with employers. These solutions are now available in many industries to keep employees engaged, safe, and healthy.

In our discussion with the global consulting company Mercer, they also confirmed a noticeable uptick in employers looking for new health-focused solutions, including DTx, that may lead to greater employee productivity and well-being, while also attempting to rein in rising health care costs. As it is important for employers to prevent the onset of debilitating conditions for their employees, DTx winners ultimately connect health care data to claims experiences that show improved outcomes with lower costs.

Such DTx–employer partnerships are becoming increasingly common. Livongo, the aforementioned US-based chronic disease management platform, has deployed a strategy whereby, via an intentional partnership network, it has formed bonds with employers and labor unions and was ultimately integrated into associated health plans offered to employees. At last report, Livongo had approximately 800 B2B partners and was serving 220,000 members. Even the US government's Employee Health Association, an insurance provider for federal employees, is a customer, accounting for 45,000 of Livongo's individual users. Not surprisingly, the company is aiming for triple-digit revenue growth.

When considering a potential partnership and after identifying employers' key challenges, whether financial or otherwise, DTx entrepreneurs must consider the path to monetization. Employers, unlike life sciences players with more established monetization strategies, may be willing to explore more creative DTx contracting approaches. These include pay-per-use, subscription-based models, and outcomes-based models. Employers who are open to new forms of collaboration typically aim to shift away from focusing on return on investment (ROI) and move toward a value of investment (VOI) frame of mind. The value here is the improved health and well-being of their employees.

DTx organizations should not forget that such partnerships can be complex and, much as life science organizations view DTx technologies as pathways toward reenergizing patient-clinician engagement, employers view them as a tool to drive effective employee engagement with their own health. For example, an overbearing, command-and-control approach from the employer could negatively impact employee engagement with the DTx platform, which in turn may affect the product's credibility through no fault of its own. Therefore, doing the necessary groundwork to ensure organic buy-in, adoption, and adherence on the part of both employers and employees are critical long-term success factors.

On the part of employers, there is also a lot of effort expected of them in terms of properly assessing, implementing, and scaling such interventions. To simplify this process, here are some tips for DTx innovators, based on learned experiences:

- Keep the buyers in mind when conveying the value of your proposed solution. This may involve the human resources function, which typically applies a risk-based approach to assess which DTx platform to partner with.
- Go into meetings with potential employer clients prepared with use cases and a business model ready for activation.
- Focus on a core set of solvable problems and don't stretch yourself too thin.
- Keep it simple: the targeted users are employees who may already have access to other health-related platforms or tools. Winning them over and achieving their engagement with a newly introduced program is a key metric of successful adoption and a prerequisite for value confirmation.
- Do your research to understand how the potential users work, and how digital solutions could address some of the employers' current challenges.
- Finally, keep in mind that employers frequently seek global contracts. The scalability and adaptability of your solution and value proposition approach across geographies may be important. This is not a trivial issue for behavioral-based DTx platforms that tend to be highly context specific.

Final Thoughts on Employers

Employers may take some time to decide whether and how to enter into a partnership with a DTx provider, especially given the wide variety of digital health offerings and the constraints of budget planning cycles. However, they offer to DTx innovators the speed and reach that few other channel partners do. As a majority of DTx innovation relies on behavior change mechanisms that can have extensive and comprehensive effects at scale, DTx platforms serve as increasingly viable and effective solutions for employers seeking to support employee health care and well-being.

Employers: A Partnership Example

The rise in chronic diseases in the United States, as in many other nations around the world, has snowballed into a genuine crisis faced by the health care system. More than half of US adults have at least one chronic disease, while over 27% have been diagnosed with two or more chronic diseases.[7] Diabetes, in particular, with 34 million affected adults, is estimated to cost the United States $367 billion per year in treatment costs and productivity loss, not including the additional 88 million adults who have prediabetes.[8]

Livongo developed a solution, a "personalized health program" as they call it, to help manage diabetes, focusing on patient empowerment to improve health outcomes and lower disease management costs. Specifically, it has developed a health signals platform by combining a mobile app, personalized coaching, connectivity to the cloud and other devices, and data science—providing a comprehensive and clinically validated care delivery model. A peer-reviewed study compared medical expenses of 2,261 Livongo program participants over a year to 8,741 matched individuals with diabetes who were not part of the program. The Livongo diabetes program resulted in a 22% reduction in medical spending, which translates into a US$88 saving per member per month at one year.[9]

In an important early decision that would propel Livongo's scale-up journey, the DTx company chose to focus its commercialization and channel partnership efforts on employers. It did so in part because enabling employees to access tailored health coaching programs resonated with its whole-person philosophy and platform to support people, especially those with chronic medical needs, to live better and healthier lives. It also made a strategic choice to support employers in keeping their staff in top shape, aligning both personal and corporate well-being objectives.

Livongo's partnership with Dean Foods is an example of how it works in practice and what it means to an employer's finances. Dean Foods had nearly 1,000 diabetic employees and faced medical costs in excess of $100,000 each year. Within one year of integrating the Livongo platform into its employee wellness programs, it achieved a 5% reduction in medical costs due to a 0.7 reduction in A1c and a 28% reduction in hypoglycemia. Dean Foods's return on investment for this pilot program was 1.4 times—defined as cost savings from improved clinical outcomes divided by the investment in Livongo's solution.[10] And the importance of a strong partnership was clear from the get-go—Dean Foods championed Livongo internally, observing an 86% activation rate among the targeted employees and a net promoter score (a measure of customer experience) exceeding 71 (versus the average of 12 obtained by corporate health plans). Not surprisingly, only a few months later Livongo successfully raised a $45 million in a Series C funding round and was acquired by Teladoc in 2020.[11]

Insurers: Potential Long-Term Strategic Partners

If there's one part of the health care value chain that is being disrupted more than any other, it is the private insurance market, particularly in the United States and Asia. In the pursuit of differentiation and customer loyalty, insurers are looking for ways to offer policyholders value-added services (VAS)—additional features and solutions beyond their core products. Medical second opinions, patient concierges, and telemedicine consultations are examples of such services. Recently insurers have expanded their offerings to include value-added wellness services, such as fitness trackers and customer rewards programs to encourage physical activity. In Asia, for example, some insurance policies have offered as many as 40 value-added services, including some at early stages of clinical evaluation or with limited validation of economic utility to insurers. Of note, implementing value-added services with limited clinical evidence may result in health and life insurers incurring higher per-employee expenditures with no apparent benefit to employees or employers.

Health insurance plans seem to be drawn to value-added services because many of these added features capitalize on current wellness trends. The insurance industry is embracing this trend in part because it is looking to improve its image and reverse the direction of its net promoter scores that measure customer loyalty and satisfaction, a good predictor of customer retention and business growth. Unfortunately, these scores in the insurance industry tend to be negative, meaning that more customers are "net detractors" rather than "net promoters."

Customer experience is critical for health insurers because it is one of the primary reasons why individuals renew or cancel their coverage. Every time a member uses health services, health insurers have numerous opportunities to help the member, from the initial diagnosis to the payment claim. It is a little more complicated for life insurance. A generally healthy person will typically only have two to three interactions with his or her life insurer per year. Too often, it may be limited to annual policy renewals or regulatory revisions. Expectedly, this can lead to disengagement and even irritation, especially if members' expectations for experience have been heightened through the rewarding experiences in other areas of their lives (e.g., ride-hailing, e-commerce platforms).

In a highly competitive business context, the pressure to balance monetization with an expanded offering of services that provide tangible clinical benefits is creating a fertile ground for disruption. DTx technologies represent a novel opportunity to insurers, beyond simply improving customer experiences. They can provide safe and effective solutions, improving health care outcomes for insurers' consumers and perhaps saving money. But how can insurers formalize this type of value-added service into a new business model?

One option for insurers is to provide their customers with a single platform or app that contains a variety of VAS solutions, a sort of VAS marketplace. VAS offerings have ranged from historical (e.g., medical second opinion) to wellness (e.g., fitness and step counter apps), and more recently, disease management (e.g., DTx for diabetes and cognitive conditions). Customers, on the other hand, may become confused if they are presented with multiple solutions from various vendors. If a solution proves to be effective, clients may forget that their insurance covers and frequently pays for these services. If things don't go as planned, it is usually the insurer who is blamed.

Another option is to bring all VAS solutions under one brand, that is, to rebrand under the insurer's brand and deliver a single end-to-end customer experience. Providing such a seamless customer experience necessitates insurers developing new capabilities: designing back-end systems, integrating data, managing liability and accountability, and so on. Insurers are also still learning about the range of solutions that customers expect from insurers or from independent providers, due to concerns about data privacy.

Independent of the deployment options, if a DTx organization wants to engage with an insurer as its distribution channel, an essential factor to remember is that traditionally, insurance is a risk-averse industry, particularly when it comes to partnership. Consequently, the near-term strategy for DTx solutions to be distributed as value-added services may target existing schemes and products that can be optimized through a DTx intervention (e.g., delivering more efficient and personalized health care, avoiding repeated claims from complications, etc.). This strategy also provides the possibility of evaluating the DTx's cost-effectiveness, by comparing the claims before and after intervention, at a scale based on a large user population. Therefore, an understanding of cost-effectiveness sets the stage for new collaboration models, pay-for-outcomes, or value-based payment based on clinical outcomes, thus moving away from the current fee-for-service reimbursement model.

Final Thoughts on Insurers

Partnering with insurers is a realistic option for scaling DTx deployment and should be pursued. Moving forward through this channel, DTx will be evaluated based on their influence on a specific client type and coverage benefit scheme, with the goal of improving clinical and financial outcomes as well as customer satisfaction. If a DTx partnership is cost-effective, insurers may be more than a vendor to DTx organizations; they could also be possible strategic partners in their development, distribution, and commercialization.

Insurers: A Partnership Example

Cigna, a multinational insurer, and Omada, a pioneer in digital behavior change and one of the largest providers of the Diabetes Prevention Program (DPP), have one of the industry's most well-known collaborations. Omada's diabetes program uses behavioral science techniques to assist members in managing their conditions with the support of a virtual care team and connected devices, such as a blood glucose meter or continuous glucose monitoring sensor.

Omada presented data from a randomized clinical trial involving almost 600 participants in 2020. One group was assigned to the Omada digital DPP program, while the other group attended traditional in-person sessions. Participants in Omada's program observed an average reduction in HbA1c of 0.23% at 12 months, compared to 0.15% in the comparison group. Also, Omada participants achieved an average weight loss of 5.4% one year after enrollment, compared to 2% weight loss in the comparison group. Overall, the study demonstrated that their digital diabetes prevention program was as effective as in-person sessions.[12]

Cigna and Omada's partnership started in 2015 when Omada began working with just a few of Cigna's self-insured employers. They have steadily broadened their collaborations since then. As a nonexclusive partner, Cigna led Omada's US$50 million funding round in 2017. Cigna wanted to shift its business toward an outcomes-based financing structure that aligned well with Omada's pay-for-performance model.

During a pilot run in 2018 between the two partners and many large employer clients, Omada's solution enabled the participants' sustained weight loss of up to 5%, a 9% drop in medical costs, and an overall ROI of 2:1. Participants also reduced their risk for type 2 diabetes by 30%, a disease for which insurers typically pay claims of US$17,000 per person per year.

TeleX Organizations: The New Front Door

TeleX, a catch-all term for telehealth, telemedicine, and telecare organizations, is widely seen as an entryway to modernizing the delivery of health care and making it more convenient for both patients and physicians. Many health care systems are dated, inefficient, and not as cost-effective as they could be due to gaps in care delivery. Their areas for improvement include patchy coordination between levels of care and challenges around patient access that are neither acceptable from a customer experience standpoint, nor fit-for-purpose from outcomes-based assessments. TeleX traditionally has three basic modalities: synchronous and asynchronous patient-provider interaction, as well as remote patient monitoring. It promises to improve patient ease and access to health care, as well as quality of service and patient satisfaction. In short, telehealth promotes the development and deployment of innovative health care delivery methods.

Despite the great potential and many successful teleX models, platforms, and prototypes, there was substantial resistance to teleX adoption prior to the COVID-19 pandemic. With the overburdening of health care facilities and restrictions on physical access to health care mediated by the coronavirus crisis, even the most tele-resistant providers warmed to the implementation of teleX solutions. In addition, regulatory barriers have been coming down for telehealth, enabling greater access and reimbursement. In the United States, 22 states changed laws or policies during the pandemic to require more robust insurance coverage of telemedicine.[13] The Centers for Medicare & Medicaid Services also expanded telehealth codes for the 2021 physician fee schedule. Privacy concerns, for better or worse, are also relaxing as populations are seeing the advantage of sharing data in return for greater protection and health system navigation.

In 2021, telehealth utilization has been 38 times higher than before the pandemic, which in turn has translated to a market share increase from around 11% prepandemic to nearly 50% at present for teleX platforms and services.[14] According to a recent McKinsey & Company report, doctors were able to see up to 175 times more patients than they did before. Three out of four teleX users reported high satisfaction, and over 50% of doctors reported having adopted a more positive attitude toward teleX since the pandemic began.[15] Exemplifying this upward trend for teleX solutions, Teladoc, a US telemedicine and virtual health care company, had over 10.6 million visits in 2020 (+156% year on year).[16] In China, Ping An Good Doctor, a leading online health care services platform, increased by 23.9% year on year their average daily consultations, to 903,000 times per day.[17] These figures confirm that the response to the COVID-19 pandemic accelerated growth in tele-health and virtualization of care pathways. An increasing number of brick-and-mortar health care organizations made the shift to virtual consultations, remote monitoring, personalized health records, and e-prescriptions as part of their own digital transformation efforts. These pre- and post-pandemic trends, together with the change in the regulatory attitude toward teleX, indicate that this important domain is likely here to stay. With that, opportunities for creative partnership are growing, too.

DTx and teleX companies are seeking to virtualize care pathways. Specifically, they are focused on delivering more person-centered care that is closer in time and space to patient needs, collecting patient-reported and biometric data that enable real-time insights for physicians, and so on. It is worth exploring partnerships in which offerings are complementary. For example, in 2020, Pear Therapeutics and UpScript Health, which provides a direct-to-consumer telemedicine platform, partnered to deliver a solution for chronic insomnia. This integrated solution includes a 10-minute telemedicine consultation with a licensed UpScript doctor to confirm if Somryst (the Pear Therapeutics DTx intervention) is appropriate for the patient. If so, the prescription is sent directly to the patient's phone, allowing them to download and access the app. Patients pay US$45 for the appointment with the doctor and, if they decide Somryst is right for them, the cost of the program will be an out-of-pocket expenditure.[18] In this scenario, not only are Pear's platform and Up-Script complementary, but teleX is also a DTx enabler. (Before this book's publication, Pear Therapeutics began a reorganization.)

Another value proposition that teleX–DTx partnerships represent is the opportunity to reach and enroll users that historically have been out of reach for traditional health care players. reach52, a Singapore-based social enterprise whose goal is to digitally reach the 52% of the global population without health care, focusing exclusively on such last mile, rural health access. As the company's CEO, Edward Booty, shares with us, "Most wealthy populations are on version 10+ of the Android operating system. reach52 deals with communities and users on version 6, which is over a decade old."[19]

While reach52 has thus far served as a "platform of platforms" for mainstream products to run health campaigns and offer access to medicines and insurance plans, the company envisions incorporating digitally delivered therapeutics into its portfolio. It hopes this will help it overcome many of the supply chain, cost, and scalability challenges startups like it typically face. Alongside its enterprising, socially responsible health care approach, the company also seeks to improve the digital maturity of the workers and communities it reaches so that digital health solutions become more acceptable and adoptable.

Final Thoughts on TeleX

As health care progressively virtualizes, there are numerous opportunities for DTx and teleX companies to collaborate. DTx can leverage the rising ecosystem adoption of teleX to reach a large user base. DTx provides clinically established solutions that extend beyond initial consultations. TeleX companies can capitalize on this opportunity to offer new products or services and build stronger relationships with patients.

Finally, teleX can be inspired by the clinical validation practices of DTx, and DTx can learn from teleX about scalability through regulation, clinician engagement, and technology integration considerations, such as data protection.

TeleX: A Partnership Example

In August 2020, US-based diabetes management DTx company Livongo was acquired for $18 billion by telehealth giant Teladoc. The union of the two companies created a $38 billion global powerhouse that provides virtually hosted health services in 175 countries across 450 medical subspecialties. Livongo has over 700 million data points on diabetes treatment trends, while Teladoc is the "world leader in whole-person virtual care."[20]

The deal was called the "biggest digital health deal ever"[21] and a "transformational opportunity to improve the delivery, access, and experience of healthcare for consumers."[22] It offers two interesting opportunities. First and foremost is the opportunity it represents for patients to experience the next generation of health care, including DTx. It represents the possibility of a more data-driven and personalized approach, providing a seamless consumer experience through the continuum of care.

Second, it opens a new cross-selling potential for both organizations. Initial research indicated just 25% overlap between Livongo and Teladoc clients across health plans, employers, and other channels. The potential to cross-sell in a DTx–telehealth partnership outweighed the potential risks and enabled the combined entity to be relevant to a broader user base with a more holistic solution set. After completing the acquisition in just three months, Teladoc has announced major deals, gaining momentum on cross-selling potential. While validation studies and establishing evidence of clinical benefits are ongoing, analysts believe such teleX–DTx initiatives will facilitate the provision of outcomes-based care that our health systems need.

Telcos: A Long-Term Outlook

Wedged between teleX and Big Tech companies is an often overlooked but highly relevant DTx channel partner: telecommunications companies (telcos). And they are everywhere—providing the connection networks over which we communicate, the phones in our hands, internet access, content streaming, and so on. Because they are so ubiquitous, telco players cannot escape the fate of any class of products or services that are readily available. They are converging on features, quality, and price, which are eventually leading to a race to the bottom in terms of profits. Faced with a downward trend in core revenues, they are at risk of being seen as pure utilities players. So, to avoid acquiring such a mundane image, and awakened to the realization that they need new markets and revenue streams, many of them are viewing the explosion of virtualized health care as an attractive opportunity.

To make the most of that opportunity, telcos need to undergo their own digital transformation first. In recent years, they have been investing heavily in developing and integrating 5G connectivity, cloud platforms, artificial intelligence (AI) capabilities, and a host of digital services. Nine of the world's largest telcos, including China Mobile, a leading telecommunications services provider in mainland China, have already adopted open application programming interfaces (APIs)—made publicly available to software developers—for digital service management.[23]

Telcos tend to be regional brands with established levels of trust, credibility, and government relations. They are also local employers that are often summoned to support the development of information technology infrastructure of health care systems and organizations. The general perception is that telcos, relative to Big Tech, are more attentive to and compliant with data privacy and security regulations, and this is definitely an advantage from the perspective the health care industry.

We have seen this favorable predisposition play out for a few telecommunications companies. In the United Kingdom over the last two decades, the BT Group has established important partnerships with the National Health Service (NHS). These include the 10-year NHS Spine contract to develop systems and software to support more than 899,000 registered users. In Australia in 2018, telco giant Telstra secured a $220 million government contract to build the National Cancer Screening Registry.[24] During the COVID-19 pandemic in South Korea, the country's three major telcos—SK Telecom, KT Corp, and LG—joined forces with the country's health care industry to enable contactless care that was strongly recommended as part of social distancing measures. Other telco–health care integration efforts in South Korea have included personalized digital health management services over the cloud, patient meal archiving through mobile phone pictures, and health trackers in nursing homes.[25]

As the experience in Korea shows, telcos can "host" entities in need of agile infrastructure solutions by fostering a marketplace of innovative service bundles and offering access to different target segments: individuals or organizations. This may mean that telcos are vendors of infrastructure first and channel partners second.

What does this mean for DTx companies in search of channel partners? While some DTx organizations may view telcos purely as B2C distributors (i.e., facilitating app downloads over the telco network), others consider them strategically positioned to support a B2B2C, "sell-with" approach to commercialization—that is, finding the right partner with the right solution to better serve the needs of end users. For example, because telcos can use their networks to aid in the management of patients with chronic disease by sending early warning signals to physicians or family members, conceptually they can play a key role in preventing avoidable complications and keeping people out of hospitals. Further, once a partnership is formed, telcos can leverage their existing arrangements with corporate customers to raise awareness about DTx solutions.

Regarding the commercial arrangement that is best suited to a DTx–telco channel partnership, a subscription-based model for access to the DTx is most likely to be the default choice for telcos. DTx innovators whose commercial gains in such a partnership would necessarily be tied to those of their counterpart must know that the fees telcos can charge are often set by the government. Therefore, profits will have an inherent limit to growth. Both sides must be flexible and inventive in their commercial models. Telcos are generally trusted providers, though this varies by country, so reputational risk in partnerships is frequently a top decision criterion for them, which is often influenced by having a validated business model and a solid vision for data play.

Final Thoughts on Telecos

Some telecom companies are just considering entering health care, while others, such as KT Corp, are already there. They have made the necessary investments to secure a long-term presence in the health care ecosystem. Telcos, like insurers, will need to demonstrate their ability to add value to solutions and services that drive clinical and efficiency gains, such as those provided by DTx organizations. Synergies between telcos and DTx developers, as well as the feasibility of such partnerships, must be rigorously evaluated with due diligence and understanding of the regulatory contexts and pathways to impact at scale. In the short- to medium-term, telcos are probably better positioned to serve as an enabler to DTx organizations.

Telcos: A Partnership Example

Our case study here is the experience of Sibel Health, a US-based spin-off from Northwestern University that specializes in biosensors used in intensive care units. They received the Spinoff Prize[26] for developing flexible devices to monitor heart rate and blood pressure in premature babies without the need of adhesive patches, which may harm a baby's delicate skin. Using their sensor technology, they launched a tracking and monitoring system of all essential vitals of COVID-19 patients in the United States and around the world.

If we are not in the DTx space, we can always learn from adjacent sectors and solutions. You may be wondering why or how a medical device company like Sibel would collaborate with and leverage any telco capabilities, but they did announce a collaboration with KT Corp, South Korea's largest telecommunications provider, in 2020.

KT aspires to be the leader in the crossing worlds of 5G, the Internet of Things (IoT), and blockchain technologies, rather than just South Korea's telecom leader. In a nutshell, they want to be the world-leading digital platform company.[27] KT was eager to expand and provide additional customer services for COVID-19-related needs. They chose to partner with Sibel to strengthen its capabilities in AI and big data–based digital health. A pilot project is now underway to assess the viability of deploying ICU-based remote monitoring services in developing countries.

KT had previously developed a Global Epidemic Prevention Platform, which alerts travelers to epidemic outbreaks and provides relevant information while tracking their movements to help prevent disease spread. In 2020, KT received funding from the Bill and Melinda Gates Foundation for a Next Generation Surveillance Study for Epidemic Preparedness, as well as a grant from the Korea-based RIGHT Fund to assist in measuring the risk of COVID-19 infection.

With KT's innovative infrastructures, and Sibel's advanced biointegrated sensors, both organizations want to "unlock the potential of AI and Big Data for the COVID-19 pandemic management and beyond."[28] The collaboration between KT and Sibel is just the beginning. Telco companies are making a bigger push into health care, and they're seeking potential partners like established and aspiring DTx organizations to quickly build capability and differentiation in the markets.

Big Tech: Potential Enablers

The opportunities for channel partnerships with diverse segments of health care actors that we have discussed so far have hopefully piqued DTx innovators' curiosity and encouraged them to seriously consider and weigh their options. Now let's turn our attention to the elephant in the room—Big Tech. It is no secret that Amazon, Apple, Facebook, and Google have a ravenous appetite for getting into the health care space, and their success in the customer experience game—coupled with their enormous cash reserves—position them as serious players over the coming decades. A wave of partnerships, acquisitions, and infrastructure build-out is already under way and likely to continue.

Kodak, the well-known photography brand, is an interesting example of this trend. Some may refer to it as "the original Big Tech player." They invented and revolutionized photography. Unfortunately, Kodak's story and downfall is almost as well-known as their cameras. After filing for bankruptcy protection in 2012 following 130 years of operations, the company saw its shares surge by 1,500% eight years later, in July 2020, when it announced a strategic pivot into pharmaceuticals. Kodak will use its extensive technology experience in chemicals and materials manufacturing to produce active pharmaceuticals ingredients, of which only 10% are manufactured in the United States today.[29] Kodak's story demonstrates the hidden opportunities the health care industry holds for established but imaginative technology brands that are willing to leverage their strengths in new ways.

In Asia, groups such as AliHealth (a subsidiary of Alibaba) and Ping An Good Doctor (a spin-off of Ping An) are following a similar trajectory. Ping An, originally a traditional insurance company, is widely known today as a financial tech and health tech player. It has over US$200 billion in cash reserves (more than double those of Amazon), over 200 million retail customers, and over 500 million internet users.[30] The company reinvests 1% of its revenues into research and development to expand its technology businesses, particularly in the areas of AI, blockchain, and cloud computing. Ping An Good Doctor, the one-stop-shop health care services platform of Ping An, has close to 70 million monthly active users who account for approximately 700,000 daily telehealth consultations.[31] When the company went public on the Hong Kong stock exchange in 2019, it raised US$1.1 billion. Its business model, based on one customer, one account, multiple products, and a one-stop shopping platform appears to be its recipe for scalability—other tech players likely have their own recipes and secret sauces too.[32]

In a sense, Big Tech companies represent a gateway to other channel partners rather than standalone partners themselves, so in order for DTx innovators to capitalize on the market power they bring, it is important that they understand the most common business models under which Big Tech operates. They don't tend to copromote any particular solution on their platforms but instead facilitate connections between potential customers and potential solutions. This is in part because the Big Tech industry has been built around the philosophy of "self-serve," which on the one hand aligns with the general vision of DTx innovators in terms of being self-driven. On the other hand, Big Tech behemoths are mostly interested in being in the business of cloud and data management, so they are often agnostic to the rationale of particular technologies that make use of their infrastructure. Big Tech can thus help DTx ventures with such strategies as setting up architecture in a cost-efficient manner and accommodating localization needs, such as data compliance and language processing.

Many of the Big Tech players offer marketplaces too. DTx solutions can be presented in these settings to drive searchability as well as interaction with the user community. In addition, these solutions can be paid for based on pay-per-use, pay-by-payers, or pay-by-employer models. Amazon, for example, has already seen a rise in genomics-related offerings and disease algorithms being managed on Amazon Web Services. This setup has certain advantages compared to DTx collaborations with more traditional partners, such as pharma companies that require an advanced level of clinical validation to be completed on both sides before engaging in discussions. On the other hand, Big Tech organizations tend to follow a shared responsibility model in which they guarantee data security while the DTx venture takes ownership of data validity.

Big Tech's forays into health care haven't all been successful. Amazon's first foray into the health sector was a 1999 investment in Drugstore.com, an online retailer of health and beauty products. Although Amazon was ahead of its time, e-prescriptions and e-pharmacies were still in their infancy and the venture was not successful. For the 2018 fiscal year, Amazon collaborated with Berkshire Hathaway and JPMorgan Chase to launch the venture Haven. Three years later, the company that was founded to disrupt US health care was shut down. The combined 1.2 million employees of the founding companies were insufficient to wring lower prices from providers and shift to a capitation model—a fixed amount paid to physicians for each enrolled person, per period of time, whether or not that person seeks care. In addition, the company's internal priorities diverged, causing it to close in early 2021.

Amazon is not the first company to fail in its attempt to disrupt health care. Remember that Google announced in 2011 that it would discontinue its personal health record platform due to scaling issues. Google's health division was then dismantled 10 years later, in 2021.

The same week, Apple confirmed that one of its most ambitious health care projects, HealthHabit, an internal application that Apple employees can use to track fitness goals, communicate with clinicians, and manage hypertension, would be scaled back. Big Tech companies are not omnipotent. Teaming up with these prominent and well-established institutions does not guarantee the venture's success.

Final Thoughts on Big Tech

Tech giants have made substantial contributions toward modernizing the health care industry. However, our previous examples have shown that the pathway between ideation and adoption can be fraught with obstacles. Disruptive technologies are insufficient on their own to disrupt a complex and fragmented industry like health care. To solve patient problems in health care, unique domain expertise that is seamlessly integrated is required, with a focus on the patient's experience rather than solely the validation of the technology. This is where DTx organizations can contribute, by leveraging emerging technologies as foundations for implementation, adoption, and scalability.

Whether it be incumbent or emerging Big Tech players, their motivations, financial resources, and infrastructural breadth and depth still represent an attractive channel partnership opportunity for DTx innovators. As DTx entrepreneurs ponder such collaborations, however, they should remain mindful of how to best pair an emerging tech platform with the established infrastructures and resources of large tech organizations in order to best position both parties for a win-win outcome.

Big Tech: A Partnership Example

As discussed in this section, the mechanism of a DTx–Big Tech partnership is often one of Big Tech companies offering the infrastructure, platform, and data capabilities necessary to propel a DTx or startup DTx innovation to greater scalability. This was the case for US- and Singapore-based Savonix, a neurocognitive assessment mobile app used to screen, track, and evaluate brain health, particularly as it pertains to possible early-stage impairments related to Alzheimer's disease and other cognitive health conditions.

Inspired by the Apple Heart Study, which was set up in 2017 in collaboration with Stanford University to analyze heart data recorded by Apple Watches and iPhones and identify irregular heart rhythms, in 2019 Boston University School of Public Health partnered with Savonix to conduct a first-of-its-kind population health study in dementia, known as the Alzheimer's Disease Discovery Study (ASSIST). The study sought to digitally collect health and lifestyle data from 400,000 people, asked them to complete a short health history questionnaire, and administered a Savonix Mobile cognitive test to assess cognitive function. The collaboration's goal was to identify differences at the personal level that could lead to the development of future interventions and treatments, such as lifestyle interventions that could be used to better prevent or manage Alzheimer's disease, in addition to genetic factors.

For the study, no doctor visits or brain scans were needed, but study participants were required to have an iPhone in order to be included in the study. They were enrolled online and asked to download the Savonix mobile app and take a series of its cognitive tests. In addition, they were asked to share exercise, nutrition, and sleep data from the iPhone Health app.

This collaboration was enabled by participation from Apple. The clinical outcome of the partnership is not known yet, but the potential is high it can lead to the development of targeted therapies for Alzheimer's disease by looking holistically across population demographics and multidimensional health factors.[33] Of note, Savonix didn't stop there and is keeping the Big Tech channel partnerships moving while the ASSIST study is recruiting participants. In 2020, they announced a partnership with Fujitsu Connected Technologies Limited, one of Japan's largest smartphone manufacturers. Savonix Mobile, the digital cognitive testing app, has been preinstalled on over a million of their Raku-Raku smartphones. The phone also includes a pedometer and other important preinstalled health care applications to support and manage the users' health.

The case study of Savonix shows how tech giants can act as an enabler, like Apple, as well as strategic partner, like Fujitsu in this case, in the distribution of digital health and DTx solutions.[34]

Conclusion

The timing has never been better for DTx innovators to seek out channel partners as a path to commercialization. While such collaborations are not required for DTx companies to succeed, the challenges associated with going the commercialization journey alone can be tough, and even insurmountable. Hence, we would suggest evaluating the likely upsides and risks involved in taking the partnership route on the road to wide-scale adoption. The good news is that the list of prospective channel partners is long and growing, given the keen interest in the health care sector by various market players expanded by the COVID-19 pandemic. From pharma to telcos to insurers, as well as newly emerging potential players, global enthusiasm toward innovation in the health care industry is at an all-time high. There are a variety of channel partner types, with respective strengths and weaknesses, for DTx innovators to explore. Or go it alone, should the circumstances allow.

Having a multipronged commercialization strategy and being prepared to pivot swiftly will probably be needed, especially in an industry such as health care, which is frequently being disrupted. As discussed earlier in the book, the most important element is keeping the problem your DTx solution is addressing as your true north during such twists. As long as decisions and course-corrections do not deviate your team from solving an established challenge, it is likely to be the most direct way to success. In short, remember to stay centered for the journey ahead.

As far as developing DTx technologies that do solve health-related challenges, we also cannot emphasize enough the importance for innovators to keep a steady focus on the heart of the matter: clinician, patient, and caregiver engagement. Many DTx innovators will have had some level of interactions with clinicians during concept validation and prototyping, but as they advance through the later stages of securing a channel partner and getting their product on the market, they may lose sight of the user experience—and that would be a mistake.

Maintaining a positive user-DTx experience—the "last mile" from a care journey and health systems perspective—is where the different strands of the DTx go-to-market journey merge together. Clinical validation, commercialization, and channel partnerships must ultimately all lead to that goal.

Just as these potential partners can be expected to scrutinize DTx solutions for commercial viability, so too should DTx innovators carefully assess their respective go-to-market channels with a view to achieving market longevity and sustainability. With so much at stake on both sides, it is understandable why such mutual "business partnership due diligence" must be performed. Based on our interviews with experts collaborating with DTx organizations, a summary of the key factors that DTx organizations would do well to consider when evaluating a potential channel partnership is found in table 11.2.

Table 11.2. Key factors to consider as part of DTx's business partnership due diligence

Strategic fit	Operational fit
• Is the partner's portfolio of offerings and data complementary to yours? • Is there an alignment with the partner in the markets (demographic or geographic) being targeted? • Is there a clear, mutually aligned, and measurable definition of success for partnership?	• Can the partner provide the necessary front-office resources (e.g., sales, marketing, access, pricing, regulatory, and medical)? • Can the partner provide the necessary supply and distribution channels? • Is the partner able to influence end users, clinicians, and administrators? In other words, does it have sufficient experience in health care or in the therapeutic area of interest to the DTx venture?
Financial fit	Cultural fit
• Is there alignment on the monetization model and flexibility therein? • Does the partner have access to sufficient capital resources and incentives? • Are both parties clear on how the partnership could evolve (e.g., mergers and acquisitions)?	• Do both parties share a common vision and mission for health care? • Does the partner have an acceptable risk and timeline tolerance? • Does the partner place emphasis on people and innovation development?

To support DTx innovators in making the right choice when selecting channel partners, and attending to the factors outlined in table 11.2, we leave you with the following recommendations:

- *Choose the right partners.* Perform your own due diligence on the readiness, willingness, abilities, and cultural fit of the prospective collaborators.
- *Conduct discovery.* Explore what matters to potential channel partners in terms of priorities, growth, unique selling propositions, challenges to overcome, and customer base.
- *Set goals and commit.* Create a plan with objectives, target markets, strategy, roles and responsibilities, resourcing, and a realistic ROI.
- *Facilitate introductions.* Invest in the relationship, assign a dedicated partner manager, and ensure continual feedback about the latest product and market developments.
- *Enable the partners.* Provide technical product training, relevant domain expertise, and sales guidance, paying special attention to those partners contributing toward a majority of the partnership.
- *Support the sales, transparently.* Ensure that pipelines and pitching opportunities are shared between partners, jointly overcoming any roadblocks and embedding customer success as a continuous improvement activity.
- *Evolve the program.* Conduct and monitor surveys, net promotor scores, reflections, and regular joint strategic planning sessions to stay aligned and ensure focus on the right set of activated channel partners.

Seek out win-win partnerships—potentially transformational for not only DTx organizations but also all partners and ecosystem stakeholders, including patients, and especially those channels that are likely to result in long-term change in health care practice and delivery. This is especially true at the time of accelerated growth of digital health, when there is a bit of a gold rush for digital applications in health care; for DTx startups and their channel partners to make a difference, the entire ecosystem (patients, clinicians, policymakers, regulators) must be aligned for the ride ahead.

What can innovative DTx companies expect in return for all this strategic evaluation and partnering? Accelerated growth, greater brand awareness, expansion of revenue potential, and new markets are all potential outcomes. We explore how to effectively articulate the value of your DTx in the next chapter.

Key Takeaways

- As DTx innovators prepare to take their solution to market, the scalability and sustainability of the company's commercialization efforts will likely require channel partnerships.
- There is a variety of channel partnership models available, traditional as well as novel, and companies must analyze which modality is most compatible with their product, end user, and business objectives.
- While DTx is a new and evolving space within health care, there are already sufficient real-world examples of both successes and failures that can serve as guideposts for entrepreneurs and help them avoid costly mistakes.

NOTES

1. Staton, "The Top 10 Patent Losses of 2015."
2. Sanofi, "Sanofi and Abbott Partner to Integrate Glucose Sensing and Insulin Delivery Technologies to Help Change the Way Diabetes Is Managed."
3. Singapore News Center, "Zuellig Pharma Shapes the Future of Healthcare with the Cloud."
4. Akili Interactive, "Akili and Shionogi Announce Strategic Partnership to Develop and Commercialize Digital Therapeutics in Key Asian Markets."
5. Organisation for Economic Co-operation and Development, "Employment Rate."
6. Centers for Disease Control and Prevention, "Workplace Health Promotion: Depression Evaluation Measures."
7. Boersma, Black, and Ward, "Prevalence of Multiple Chronic Conditions among US Adults, 2018."
8. Centers for Disease Control and Prevention, *National Diabetes Statistics Report 2020: Estimates of Diabetes and Its Burden in the United States.*
9. Whaley et al., "Reduced Medical Spending Associated with Increased Use of a Remote Diabetes Management Program and Lower Mean Blood Glucose Values."

10. Dean Foods and Livongo Health, *Livongo Drives 1.4x ROI in Year 1 for Dean Foods.*

11. Landi, "Telehealth Leader Teladoc to Buy Livongo in $18.5B Deal."

12. Omada Health, "Omada Digital Diabetes Prevention Program Shows Sustained HbA1c Reduction and Weight Loss in Randomized Control Trial."

13. Volk et al., "States' Actions to Expand Telemedicine Access during COVID-19 and Future Policy Considerations."

14. Bestsennyy et al., "Telehealth: A Quarter-Trillion-Dollar Post-COVID-19 Reality?"

15. Bestsennyy et al., "Telehealth."

16. Landi, "Teladoc's Virtual Visits Reach 3M during Q4 as Revenue Grows to $383M."

17. Ping An, *2020 Annual Report*, 65.

18. UpScripts Somryst, "Train your Brain for Better Sleep."

19. From an interview with the authors, September 17, 2021.

20. Teladoc Health, "Teladoc Health to Announce Third Quarter 2022 Financial Results."

21. Forrester, "The Biggest Digital Health Deal of All Time: Teladoc and Livongo."

22. Teladoc Health, "Teladoc Health and Livongo Merge to Create New Standard in Global Healthcare Delivery, Access and Experience."

23. TM Forum, "Telco Cloud Orchestration Plus, Using Open API on IoT."

24. STL Partners, "Four Strategies for Telcos in Healthcare."

25. Yonhap, "Telcos Expand Digital Health Care Services amid Pandemic."

26. "Scailyte among the Spinoff Finalists for the Global Nature Research Awards," Swiss Biotech.

27. KT Corporation, "S.Korea's KT Corp. to Expand Digital Health Business with Sibel."

28. Koh, "KT Signs MoU with Sibel Health to Expand Its Digital Health Capabilities."

29. Blankenship, "Camera Maker Kodak Dives into Drug Manufacturing with $765M Federal Loan."

30. Ping An, *Announcement of Unaudited Results for the Three Months Ended March 31, 2020.*

31. Ping An, "Ping An Good Doctor Has Become the First Online Healthcare Platform with More Than 300 Million Registered Users."

32. Ping An, "Ping An Unveils Health Care Ecosystem Strategy."

33. Savonix, "Savonix and Boston University School of Public Health Launch Landmark Population Health Alzheimer's Disease Discovery Study (ASSIST) to Digitally Collect Brain Health Data."

34. Savonix, "Savonix and Fujitsu Connected Technologies Limited Partner to Introduce Savonix Mobile App on Raku-Raku Smartphone F-42A."

The Price Is Right

Value in the Eye of the Beholder

As we have seen through the multitude of real-world examples provided so far in this book, the health care industry is slowly pivoting toward a value-based model in which reimbursement is increasingly tied to patient health outcomes rather than to the volume of products and services delivered. DTx technologies and companies are well-placed to accelerate this shift through better data collection and cost-effective, consumer-friendly platforms. For this reason, DTx innovators must have a pricing strategy in place that serves not only to engage potential channel partners but also to reflect the role their solutions play in bringing legacy health systems and operations up to speed with evolved expectations around value-based care. The question of pricing, therefore, lies in successfully conveying the value they bring to those partnerships and to the payer.

DTx monetization, especially in relation to reimbursement, is a new and complicated topic. It is considered one of the key impediments to DTx adoption. Addressing a pathway to reimbursement, if applicable, should be considered early on. Not only must DTx entrepreneurs take the time to understand the motivations of their potential channel partners, but they should also identify payers and their dynamics in

Table 12.1. DTx commercial models in the United States

Archetype	Reimbursement	Minimum requirements		
		FDA clearance	Prescription	Clinical evidence
Business to consumer	Cash pay	No	No	No (highly recommended)
Business to business	Providers (hospitals, practices), pharma, or medtech	No	No	Usually (highly recommended)
Business to payer	Programmatic spending	No	No	Usually (highly recommended)
	Claims-based reimbursement	Yes	Yes	Yes

Source: Hoult, "Key Factors to Obtaining Reimbursement for Digital Therapeutics in the US."

the health care industry. Payers, which may be public or private, are entities that will cover the cost of the service provided by the DTx to the end users. DTx innovators should explore all possible reimbursement pathways that may be available to them through both types of the payers while also seeking to understand the range of engagement models for each payer (table 12.1).

The first step toward developing a value-based offering is to define what "value" is and how it will be measured. DTx organizations should collaborate with their channel partners to reach an alignment in this area as each stakeholder has its own incentives and metrics by which it assesses value and makes decisions. DTx platforms that simultaneously satisfy multiple parties have a higher chance of achieving commercial success.

Providers typically consider something to be of value based on the appropriateness of care and effective, evidence-based interventions. Meanwhile, patients value health services or interventions if they lead to clinical improvement and better functional health and provide user experiences that are as seamless and minimally invasive (both surgically and practically) as possible with minimal or no disruption to their personal, professional, and social lives. From health care managers' perspectives, value could also be defined as the clinical benefits and health improvements achieved for the money spent. To paraphrase a familiar saying, value is in the eye of the beholder.

Which of these value definitions should be the focus of a DTx offering? The answer depends on the deployment context and channel partners and may incorporate several value definitions tailored to the business model. Let us take a closer look at the payers as well as some potential factors to consider when determining DTx value.

Public Payers: A Focus on the Evidence

Most health care systems around the world are publicly financed in some way, meaning that reimbursement through the state is or should be a key consideration for any DTx commercial strategy. Public payers' awareness of DTx has grown significantly in recent years. Some initially provided access to digital health apps and DTx as part of programmatic spending for wellness and disease management. Others have been slow to adopt new technologies or adapt their payment methodologies to cover DTx. Many public payers now have or are thinking about establishing a digital health formulary. Regardless of the country where DTx organizations operate, and the archetype of commercial models, public payers will consider regulatory submission, clinical data, and health economics outcomes for potential coverage as well as the payment level at which they will reimburse. Put it simply, DTx organizations must demonstrate that their products are medically necessary.

While going the fully validated, regulated route to commercialization may seem like a daunting, time-consuming, and costly exercise for DTx innovators, this is the way translational science—the process of applying knowledge and insights from basic science and clinical trials to techniques, tools, and interventions that address critical medical needs—operates. Robustly addressing this pathway differentiates DTx platforms from nonregulated digital health solutions. This is a must for the "golden ticket": securing claims-based reimbursement at scale. Arguably, it is one of the most difficult paths to achieve in the context of bringing a product to market, since the arduous and necessary process of clinical validation alone may not be sufficient for commercial success. More specifically, this space also requires DTx organizations to spend considerable time and effort demonstrating the economic need for and efficacy of new treatments, and obtaining robust evidence to support such claims is frequently done on a limited budget.

Most importantly, DTx innovators must be aware of the chasm between approval and reimbursement. Regulatory clearance, such as approval from the Food and Drug Administration (FDA), does not guarantee that any payor will provide reimbursement. Data needed to clear the FDA are often insufficient for coverage and market adoption. There is a long list of novel medical technologies that are in "funding purgatory," which means they have been approved as clinically sound but do not have a clear coverage model in terms of who pays for them. This again underscores the importance of having a reimbursement road map as part of a DTx company's go-to-market strategy. Some may argue that coverage pathways should be considered only if and when marketing approval is obtained. In our view, given how important this aspect is for DTx sustainability and integration into the broader health system, formulating a vision and an action plan as soon as feasibly possible is a differentiating advantage for serious innovators. That is why clinical studies should be designed not just to demonstrate the safety and efficacy of a solution but also to address payers' potential concerns. Payers are not only asking for outcomes data but long-term data as well. What would be the long-term value and impact of a 12-week exercise and cognitive behavioral therapy intervention program, for example? Would such digital intervention provide long-term benefits to payers? Will these benefits "stick"?

Generating data, specifically real-world evidence, needs to be a top priority. While focusing on public payers, we encourage DTx organizations to explore ways they can collaborate, early, with governmental agencies and organizations, not only to obtain an endorsement but also to collect real-world data. Singapore, for example, recently rolled out mindline.sg, a one-stop mental health platform that matches users with resources and helplines. Within that platform, it integrated Wysa, an aspiring DTx that operates an emotionally intelligent chatbot that "listens" to people's mental health struggles and anxieties and guides them to appropriate cognitive behavioral therapy or coaching exercises.

The Wysa model is illuminating because while its success relies on the government's endorsement and adoption, the company focused on gaining traction and business funding through a direct-to-consumer model first before they approached the public sector for scale. Singapore's government currently pays for the Wysa license at a discounted rate and offers the platform for free to people in the country. Outside of Singapore, and perhaps eyeing a similar B2C-to-nationwide scale-up, Wysa is also being deployed at Cincinnati Children's Hospital in the United States and at the North East London National Health System Foundation Trust in the United Kingdom.

Singapore's experience with incorporating digitally delivered mental wellness services shows that if DTx innovators aspire to broaden market adoption, they should consider what it would take to convince large payers, such as central governments or regional health boards, to adopt their solutions. Yet, all too often, DTx business and pricing propositions are based on the founders' and developers' desire to recoup their research and development investment rather than on a strong health economic model that demonstrates the potential of their technology to achieve cost savings based on improvements in patient outcomes.

Public payers cannot afford to overinvest. They may be unconvinced by revenue-prioritizing commercial models unless they clearly map out their value to the health system. To stand a chance of successfully garnering public reimbursement of their products, therefore, DTx innovators must uncover these value-return ratios and extrapolate them to the population level, showing how their solution alleviates illness, disease management, or economic and other resource allocation–related challenges. This stresses, once again, the importance of strong health economics and outcomes research to bolster a DTx product's pathway to move beyond technical and clinical validation and achieve sustained adoption.

Seeking public reimbursement is an important strategy for DTx innovators looking to scale. With this in mind and the points just mentioned, here are a few practical tips when approaching the public sector as a potential payer:

- Target major health care utilization shifts, such as the transitioning away from care delivery to health preservation, from hospitals to home, or from a focus on quality alone to the overall value that is in line with the governments' broader strategic transformation goals.
- Adapt DTx solutions (or have a plan to do so) to the local context. Governments are open to ideas from around the world, but DTx innovators must show a clear capability for localization.
- Demonstrate value not only in financial or clinical terms but also in terms of the DTx's staying power, or "stickiness," month after month—defined by how memorable, valuable and habit-forming a DTx is for any individual user so they will actually continue to use the solution on a regular basis.
- Think about the potential business models (including reimbursement) and the scalability of your DTx on a national scale early on (which is the perk of partnering with government).

Private Payers: A Focus on Returns and Value

In the aim of better price points, targeting private payers (e.g., in a business-to-business approach or programmatic spending; see table 12.1) tends to be the preferred option for DTx and aspiring DTx solutions. DTx entrepreneurs can in fact negotiate on a case-by-case basis with health insurance plans and employers. However, the potential end-user base is usually smaller than that available through nationwide coverage.

In many countries, insurance and employer benefits schemes are being revised and regulated more rigorously than in the past, both by the country or local governments and by the organizations themselves, as payers attempt to assure adequate coverage while keeping overall costs under control. As a result, private payers are increasingly offering their members health services and solutions that fall within a certain financial threshold and are therefore assessing the "price asked" by the providers of those services against the clinical and economic value they generate, as we discussed earlier. Furthermore, many private payers impose co-payments, deductibles, and other out-of-pocket expenditures, implying that not every service included in an insurance policy is necessarily fully covered and patients themselves share in the cost of care.

Because of the variability across these options in the private payer market, defining a pricing strategy for a DTx product is more complex than putting a price tag on a new medical device or therapy. In the absence of real DTx alternatives and of well-defined reimbursement mechanisms, DTx innovators, should resources allow, consider pursuing two avenues concurrently:

- *Focus on value.* DTx solutions that create measurable value for patients, providers, and payers should be priced accordingly. This includes understanding and measuring both users' perceptions of the DTx's benefits and the value it creates within and along the care continuum.
- *Focus on cost (and so, returns).* DTx entrepreneurs should be considering all the direct and indirect costs involved in developing, deploying, and distributing a DTx to their partner and end users when assessing their cost-effectiveness.

Here we turn our attention to how DTx can align their pricing models with the value they provide to patients, other health care stakeholders, and the health care system in general.

Users' Willingness to Pay

Understanding the value of a DTx technology starts with understanding its target users' willingness to pay (WTP) for the benefit it offers. This is particularly relevant in contexts where providing such solutions implies out-of-pocket expenditures. Households in countries that are part of the Organisation for Economic Co-operation and Development finance about 25% of the cost of prescription medication.[1] In the United States, it is common for patients to have a 20% co-pay or coinsurance. In these situations, a DTx pricing model must account for a key wild card—users' willingness to not only use the solution but also to pay for it. This factor is also likely to influence its uptake by providers. (If patients are not willing to pay for the solution, doctors will have little reason to prescribe it.)

Estimating potential DTx users' willingness to cover the costs of use is an important exercise DTx innovators need to undertake when developing their pricing strategy. It reveals the economic constraints within which patients are willing to consider a solution. This important exercise is truly about understanding the real value-drivers of a DTx to each cohort or customer segment, as well as these individuals' willingness to forego the intervention in place of another solution or other pressing personal expenses.[2]

A WTP analysis should also be entirely contextualized to the geography, socioeconomic status, and disease pathways of the targeted patient population. It is important that this analysis addresses the foundation of the solution—that is, what is the unmet need being solved with the solution and what impact is the solution expected to have? Such analysis is what drives the business case for channel partners and payers to engage with DTx innovators who are keen on building up their portfolio of platform play capabilities. DTx entrepreneurs should consider average income levels, discretionary spending, and health or social balance for productive living to arrive at a figure that is acceptable to the population while also remaining economically viable for DTx organizations and potential channel partners.

In a US study, for example, researchers studied participants' willingness to pay to be part of a blood pressure control study. They asked patients a series of questions about time and travel costs, as well as time value related to their study participation. They found out that the mean WTP was of $25 out of pocket for a doctor's consultation.[3] The final pricing, in our opinion, is just as important as the factors that led to the $25 price point, since it was discovered that more than 50% of patients did not have insurance coverage or a designated primary care provider. Based on findings like these, we also encourage DTx entrepreneurs to conduct a price elasticity analysis to pinpoint whether an increase or decrease in prices would generate different outcomes, such as a change in DTx consumption. How might a $30 versus a $20 consultation fee affect patients' willingness to participate in the blood pressure study and see their doctor? The same reasoning applies to DTx.

In summary, out-of-pocket payments strongly influence patient decision-making as well as physician choice when it comes to prescribing a DTx solution. Whether your DTx commercialization strategy targets public or private payers (or both), channel partners will expect a WTP analysis as part of any comprehensive distribution negotiation. This is a reminder that beyond setting a price point for their product, DTx innovators must first and foremost consider the holistic value they are offering to each of the key decision-makers involved in its uptake.

Pricing Models

When pricing their solution, innovators sometimes mistakenly believe that mimicking a pricing model for another technology-driven niche of the market, however successful (e.g., software as a service, or SaaS),[4] will also catapult this new innovation to commercial success. Transporting pricing and sales models from other sectors wholesale, however, rarely works in health care because of the myriad unique biological and organizational factors that characterize it.

In the course of our research for this book, we came across a variety of pricing model archetypes that could serve as an inspiration for DTx innovators in their discussions with private channel partners. They each have their merits relative to the industries and business contexts in which they are commonly used and, as mentioned, must be tailored not only to health care's singular context but also to the channel

Table 12.2. Popular pricing model archetypes adaptable for DTx, especially relevant in a B2C and B2B business models

One-off payment	Device and consumables
• Charge per intervention, procedure, test, or activity with reimbursement and/or out-of-pocket payment	• "Razor-razorblade" model: relevant for solutions with consumables and/or such supplies as DTx for diabetes management coming with strips, continuous glucose monitoring sensors, and/or infusion sets or accessories for the insulin pump

Subscription	Maintenance
• Pure: subscription-based, including fixed and variable components • Freemium: free basic service with optional fees for access to advanced features • Leveling: tiered customer categories based on user profiles, utilization, and features	• License: annual renewal, including technical support and software updates • Rental: applicable for hardware, on a lease with depreciation costing

partners and payers with whom DTx entrepreneurs are considering to engage on the path to commercialization. To help orient them in this process, we highlighted a few of the most popular models (table 12.2) and a list of questions whose answers should guide them in making the right choices.

Checklist of considerations for selecting the right pricing model:

❏ What are your geography, therapeutic area, and clinical and health economics outcomes data?

❏ Is the solution purely a digital offering or does it involve a companion drug, medical device, or other equipment? If so, how would DTx pricing fit into the reimbursement model of the item or device that is now reimbursed or seeks reimbursement?

❏ What is the current level of competition within the therapeutic area being addressed? Are there digital and nondigital options? Would the DTx potentially replace an existing item or service already with a high reimbursement rate?

- What is the differential advantage of the proposed DTx compared to what is already out on the market, both digital and nondigital?
- What are the potential applicable reimbursement models or archetype models as discussed earlier?
- Who is expected to pay for the product and the potential co-payment/out-of- pocket expenditures for patients?
- Who are the targeted end users and what is their willingness to pay if they are expected to bear all or part of the cost?
- What is the level of maintenance or servicing required to maintain a current iteration of the solution? How regularly does the software need to be updated?
- What could be the number of potential DTx prescriptions at scale?
- How often are patients and caregivers expected to use the DTx and for how long?

A combination of pricing strategies may often be appropriate, depending on the therapeutic area being addressed, the type of business model (B2B, B2B2C, or B2C), and the geography. For example, Blue-Star® (the diabetes management solution powered by Welldoc that was discussed in the earlier chapters of this book) offers a variety of products and their respective pricing models to different customers (i.e., employers, health plans, or health systems) in a B2B2C approach. JOGO, a US-based DTx company with international operations in Asia, leveraging wearable sensors, artificial intelligence, and virtual reality to treat neuromuscular conditions using neuroplasticity and biofeedback, is also a good example of business model and revenue diversification. The company's long-term strategy is to create a current procedural terminology code (a set of medical codes that are used by health care professionals to bill medical services and procedures to public and private health insurance programs for potential reimbursement) so JOGO can be prescribed and reimbursed. Meanwhile it is exploring three distinct revenues streams:

- *DTx as a service.* In the United States, JOGO is FDA-registered with its service covered by Medicare and commercial insurance plans. It can be delivered at clinics or via telemedicine. In India, patients typically learn about this solution through a specialist's referral from private hospital chains, which do not accept insurance. Therefore, the service is expected to be an out-of-pocket expense.
- *Revenue sharing with distribution channels.* JOGO has signed copromotion deals with large pharma and medical devices companies that have complementary products in the neuromuscular diseases therapeutic area. As part of the deal, the channel partners' salesforces are leveraged to promote the DTx along with their respective pharmaceutical compound or device.
- *Franchise model.* In India and Malaysia, JOGO has successfully piloted a franchise concept whereby doctors refer patients to a JOGO franchise, a dedicated physical clinic owned by the franchisee. In this distribution model, JOGO receives a percentage of the revenues obtained from providing the services to patients, regardless of whether these services are delivered in the clinic or remotely.

As previously stated, too, there are geographical considerations for potential DTx pricing models. We encourage DTx entrepreneurs to use the checklist provided to determine the most suitable pricing model for their solution while remaining compliant with all applicable local and federal regulations.

Whichever approach DTx entrepreneurs choose to follow, potential channel partners will expect them to bring forth a motivated pricing proposition. Channel partners can then look at their existing portfolio and leverage their knowledge of the payer ecosystem to help refine the offering in a way that works to their advantage too. DTx innovators who have done their homework and have a solid business plan, while being flexible about finding common ground, are the ones that "make us sit up in our seats," as one channel partner put it.

Therefore, it is incumbent on DTx players to get the right commercial expertise and team in place that can help them define an optimal pricing model.

Value-Based Care

Discussing DTx pricing models implies exploring value-based pricing as well. It is a closely related concept and underlying philosophy for many pricing models. Value-based pricing agreements pay providers and DTx organizations based on the quality of care they offer, focusing on improving patients' clinical outcomes (quality) rather than the volume of health care services supplied or patients treated (quantity). Although we do not attempt in this book to explain the intricacies of value-based pricing in infinite detail, as health care becomes increasingly outcome-driven, we do feel it is important for DTx innovators to understand them in broad strokes. We raise the point as well because value-based pricing has evolved beyond the classical understanding of value-based care, which shifted the focus from fee-for-service to health outcomes over cost.

The contemporary definition of "value" is not just derived from measuring health outcomes against the cost of delivering the outcomes, but it also considers factors such as the appropriateness of care given the social and individual context in which it is provided (figure 12.1).

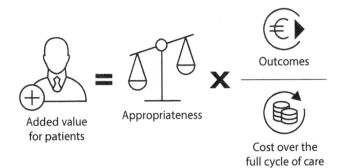

FIGURE 12.1. Defining value in health care from a patient's perspective. Source: Heuvel et al., *Pathway to Success in Outcome-Based Contracting*

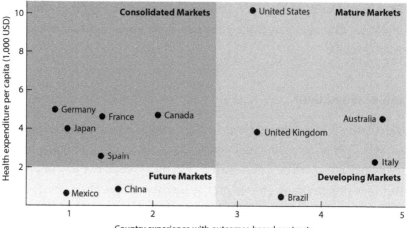

FIGURE 12.2. Country health expenditure (per capita) and experience with outcomes-based contracts (on a scale of 1 to 5, with 1 being the least experienced countries and 5 being the most experienced). Source: Heuvel et al., *Pathway to Success in Outcome-Based Contracting*, 12 (citing original figure data sources as OECD, the World Bank, Navigant, and KPMG Payer primary market research)

In line with this updated understanding of value-based care, pricing models are starting to become more nuanced and granular as well. These arrangements are actively being put in place (figure 12.2).

According to KPMG, in the United States between 2016 and 2019, the therapeutic areas of cardiology, neurology, and endocrinology accounted for more than 70% of the total outcomes-based deals between the developers of health care solutions and providers and/or payers.[5] Novartis, for example, has entered into such agreements with health care providers by pledging to pay for any treatments that may still be required beyond the 14-session standard of care for their Lucentis drug that is used to treat age-related macular degeneration. Similarly, the company's pricing with insurers for its heart failure drug, Entresto, is also based on outcomes, which are measured as the extent to which the drug improves patients' health. Novartis signed several contracting models that tie pricing to patient outcomes, such as with health insurers, like with Cigna and Aetna.

For their part, health plans are also becoming increasingly engaged in the conversation around value-based pricing. In 2017, the nonprofit health insurer Harvard Pilgrim Health Care in the United States agreed with Amgen, the pharmaceutical company, to the first cardiovascular outcomes-based refund contract. Under the contract, Amgen would issue a full rebate to the health plan if a patient continued to suffer strokes or heart attacks after a full course of treatment with its antibody therapy Repatha.[6]

While this book encourages DTx innovators to take note of such novel concepts around pricing, the industry is still fundamental in its traditional and well-established payment mechanisms. As expressed earlier, DTx teams must onboard the appropriate skills and experience to match the channel partners' and payers' expectations and arrive with business and commercial models in hand.

Conclusion

DTx pricing is the monetary reflection of its perceived (and demonstrated) value in the eye of the beholder. While the FDA focuses on such areas as DTx safety, insurers may be interested in how DTx deployment may impact claims, and patients may be interested in how the DTx solutions might help them live a healthier life for any associated out-of-pocket cost.

Earlier we emphasized the importance of demonstrating DTx safety and effectiveness alongside robust health care economics outcomes, which are collectively at the foundation of bridging innovation with commercial success. Insufficiently accounting for all of these factors, even with a powerful channel partner in place, may substantially impede or even preclude commercializing DTx platforms in the competitive health care landscape. Increasingly, evidence of effectiveness and safety in the form of real-world evidence (RWE) may be required in order for DTx platforms to be reimbursable. To generate sufficient data and RWE, some DTx organizations are going "at-risk"—being paid only if a set of predefined health outcomes are being met—via value-based and return-on-investment-based pricing models with private and public channel partners.

An example of this approach was employed by Hello Heart, a DTx focused on blood pressure management, to demonstrate that its platform could successfully lower user blood pressure with outcomes-based compensation instead of subscription-based payment by the client.[7] Similar return-on-investment-based payment structures have also been explored by Naluri for its chronic disease management solution. These scenarios, while potentially risky for the solution provider, may also play a catalytic role in scaling adoption due to the heavy emphasis placed on payment being driven by demonstrated efficacy. Nonetheless, this reimbursement approach can be considered and is potentially effective for the community of DTx developers. When considering the broader landscape of how payers are viewing the future of DTx reimbursement, recent analysis in the insomnia space has shown that 9 out of 10 managed care organizations surveyed already have or will have DTx reimbursement plans in place. To help payers better prepare for a potential increase in DTx reimbursement activity, Express Scripts, the largest pharmacy benefit-management organization in the United States, has developed a digital health formulary to help payers systematically evaluate digital health solutions for potential coverage and offerings to members.[8]

Regarding costs, we encourage DTx innovators to spend time truly understanding the patient pathways to which their product applies, the total direct and indirect cost of care in the current model (including down to the unit and activity level, or patients' potential out-of-pocket expenses), and how incorporating a DTx solution could lead to improved health outcomes at the same or lower cost (if any).

With value, cost, and outcomes data, DTx entrepreneurs can start exploring different pricing mechanisms that might exist in their respective geographies. If leveraging the elements and building blocks of the technology industry, such as in a SaaS approach, for example, seems like the fastest way to monetize DTx, we expect (and advise) DTx to build first on traditional biopharma and medical technology companies' business and pricing models. New and hybrid models and reimbursement pathways, combined with a variety of channels (i.e., B2C and B2B2C), will emerge over time. As DTx are building evidence-based value propositions, our hope is that they not only transform the care delivered but also advance the adoption of value-based contracting schemes.

Key Takeaways

- Value is in the eye of the beholder, so DTx innovators must seek to understand potential channel partners' and payers' motivations for collaboration so as to align their proposed pricing model.
- Given the focus and expected use of their solution, DTx innovators should consider private- as well as public-sector reimbursement; this can be done in sequence or tandem.

NOTES

1. Organisation for Economic Co-operation and Development, *Out-of-Pocket Spending: Access to Care and Financial Protection.*

2. Defining the needs prioritization for each potential cohort or customer segment can be inspired by A. H. Maslow's theory of human motivation and the five categories of human needs that dictate an individual's behavior (Maslow, "A Theory of Human Motivation," *Psychological Review* 50, no. 4 (1943), 370–96, https://doi.org/10.1037/h0054346).

3. Gleason-Comstock et al., "Willingness to Pay and Willingness to Accept in a Patient-Centered Blood Pressure Control Study."

4. Software as a service, also known as "on-demand software," is a software licensing and delivery model in which software is licensed on a subscription basis and delivered via the Internet.

5. Heuvel et al., *Pathway to Success in Outcome-Based Contracting.*

6. Heuvel et al., *Pathway to Success in Outcome-Based Contracting.*

7. Henze et al., "Moving Digital Health Forward: Lessons on Business Building."

8. Prabhu and Menon, "Express Scripts a Pioneer: Launches Curated List of Digital Therapeutics."

.

The Future of DTx

This chapter was written with the contribution of Dr. Eddie Martucci, cofounder and CEO of Akili Interactive Labs in the United States.

In 2011, Eddie Martucci, cofounder of Akili Interactive Labs, was convinced that technology was the best vehicle for providing novel treatments for neurological and psychiatric diseases in ways drug-based therapies alone were not able to do. Akili was born from what Eddie perceived as a need and an aspiration for a new modality that would reimagine medicine and care delivery through software. Today, the broad modality of software addressing health conditions is a rapidly growing field that provides patients with the opportunity to experience their care in a more user-friendly, self-directed, even fun way, though no less rigorously sound than traditional treatment pathways. Akili pursued developing prescription DTx, where clinically validated therapeutic software is prescribed by doctors to treat a disease. "When we shared our vision back then, people would raise eyebrows and be quite skeptical of something like a video game interface that could be as effective as traditional medicine prescribed by a doctor," remembers Eddie.

It took more than a decade for the biopharmaceutical and medical device industry, regulators, and early DTx pioneers like Akili to grow the industry and address key "firsts" for DTx, such as product development and validation, conducting robust clinical trials with DTx software to demonstrate clinical evidence on par with traditional therapeutics, and identifying a pathway for obtaining market authorization by regulatory bodies. Those efforts have paved the way for a wave of DTx solutions that seemed like science fiction less than a decade ago but are actually being realized in the hands of patients today.

The vision and the slowly growing momentum behind DTx were elevated to near the top of the health care agenda when the COVID-19 pandemic began to wreak havoc and reveal the weaknesses of the established care models. Those models, based on physical check-ins, brick-and-mortar waiting rooms, and in-person physician consultations on the one hand, and bedeviled by challenges around treatment adherence and patient monitoring on the other, were suddenly primed for disruption. The COVID-19 crisis gave rise to new partnership opportunities and alternative solutions as patients began to cancel traditional doctor's appointments and health organizations began to offer options to access care differently—in patients' homes and communities instead of at hospitals and clinics. Many physicians and patients who may have never had a video conference call before became comfortable with telemedicine-based services and remote monitoring platforms and applications.

Similarly, and just as pervasively, nearly every family experienced some version of the stress, anxiety, and psychological issues previously relegated to diagnosed mental health conditions. Thus, COVID-19 simultaneously had a major direct impact on growing the awareness of and need for new, scalable, and accessible interventions. Enter digital options for treatment and care that, perhaps even more so than telemedicine, will be here to stay for the long term.

Digital health tools, including DTx, pharma companion apps, and wellness platforms, reached an inflection point in popularity, leading to a gold rush of experimentation by health care stakeholders. The regulatory environment adapted seemingly instantaneously, and many of the barriers that had previously held back progress in operationalizing digital health technology, such as availability, cost, and market adoption, seemed to shift overnight. In addition to drugs and durable medical devices, consumers began asking for digital treatments—and physicians are now prescribing DTx. Thanks in part to the urgency created by COVID-19, and cruising on the wings of broad digital transformation, "software as medicine" became a reality.

DTx are now poised to reimagine health care, and the future is exciting. Software-based interventions are interacting with human physiology in ways never seen before, such as incorporating music to assist with walking in people with neurological disorders, treating Alzheimer's using noninvasive light-based stimulation techniques, or losing oneself in a fun video game that is actually rewiring neural processing and treating attention dysfunction in children. If breakthroughs such as these are any indication, DTx are going to revolutionize health care and eventually be integrated into mainstream medicine. But this revolution is more than just the dawn of new medical products; we're seeing the emergence of an entirely new pillar of medicine that can engage and respond to patients in dramatically new ways, putting the role of the patient more central than ever before.

The Role of Patients in a New Era of Medicine

Patients are ready for change. They are more informed and empowered than ever before, expecting a high-end user experience in *all* aspects of their lives, and being seen not as conditions to treat but as individuals to heal. With DTx, patients like you and I, and future generations, will experience medicine differently. Many of these new technology benefits will be unobstructive to the patient and, in many cases, actually exciting (Akili, for example, has a design ethos that their treatment products are entertaining enough that, in the moment of the DTx experience, the patient might forget they are "taking medicine" at all). Indeed, DTx offer inspiration and empowerment to patients in new ways because the experiences they provide can be intentionally designed to be engaging and exciting. For instance, using virtual reality to ease pain and video game interfaces to improve ADHD impairments can be fun and captivating. Even more exciting, the patient is finally empowered to play a central role in the management of their condition by directing the management's evolution in response to digitally delivered insights, reminders, and prompts, or "nudges" in the simplest case. This empowerment is further supported by real-time product adaptations and highly personalized product features designed to allow personalized benefit.

Furthermore, the real-world data and feedback of DTx users can be of great value to DTx organizations, physicians, and care teams, as they can inform improvements to the interaction design, underlying software, and eventually disease treatment provided by these tools. In a positive turn on the "uses of data" controversy we've seen with social media platforms, companies are using data from DTx to actually enhance their products' core value proposition to patients over time, allowing an evolution of safety, effectiveness, and patient experience not only in future products but in the exact same products that are in patients' hands. The future of medicine can be rapidly adaptive, and the incentive of business and user benefit will be aligned.

A vast population of patients—more than many health care leaders and providers expect—are ready to experience new treatment modalities.[1] It is they who will own the design and evolution of the DTx ecosystem, and it is they who will eventually determine the demand for DTx. As Eddie recalls, "One of the very first days that our first product was available on the market, without any product marketing, a physician called Akili to know more about our treatment because one of her patients had already asked her twice for a prescription." Patients are activated and anticipating the new wave.

A New Patient-Physician Relationship

Although DTx are not designed to replace traditional medicine or drugs, they offer a new type of treatment modality and a new promise for patients and physicians that can be used as part of an overall treatment program, either alone or alongside traditional medicine. But do DTx threaten to replace physicians?

This question has sparked a series of long debates, but the conclusion is clearly no.[2] We see technology, and within that DTx, as quite the opposite: enablers of a better patient-physician relationship, which in itself is a key driver of clinical outcomes.[3] If technology is designed properly, it should enhance this relationship by involving other members of the clinic care team (e.g., technicians, nurses, or social workers), as well as the patients' caregivers, whose critical role is often overlooked. And technology can offer rich data to drive meaningful dialogue between patients and their physicians.

Focusing on treatment for children with ADHD, Akili developed ADHD Insight, a behavior-tracking app and online dashboard that helps parents monitor changes in their child's ADHD symptoms. Through the data and feedback collected from the children and their care teams, parents can understand how their child is doing and feeling on a daily basis. Eddie says, "We expected the first piece of parent feedback to be about the nuances of what the data means about specific symptoms, but the number one thing we hear from parents is that it's actually helping them have better conversations with their children, as well as more meaningful conversations with the physicians and their staff." This type of unexpected insights should not be overlooked: families care deeply about their relationships, perhaps more so than their specific symptoms—and digital platforms can enhance this.

Today in traditional medicine there are few data to guide such physician-patient conversations beyond the patient's memory and recollection of how they feel. In mental health, in particular, having more precise real-world data is especially relevant as it can mean the difference between continuing with the same approach to treatment, modifying it, or switching to an entirely different one. DTx can collect such data every day, or potentially many times per day. And when it's shared with physicians, patients, and the broader care team, it creates the foundation for a new type of relationship in medicine that doesn't exist today.

Evolving Business Models

The digital therapeutics landscape will evolve drastically over the next few years, with the anticipated arrival of new applications and increased reimbursement coverage by commercial health plans and government payers. In the case of specific disease treatments, DTx will continue to be prescription-based products, but our hope is that the prescribing ability of physicians will grow relative to the limitations they currently face in many countries in terms of who can prescribe what digital tool for what purpose. DTx formularies will ultimately expand and be less restricted not only because of different safety profiles compared to traditional medicine, but also because with time health care practitioners will gain a more comprehensive understanding of how these products work. Independent of formularies, as more medical practitioners get their first and second experiences prescribing DTx, the "new modality" barrier will recede and doctors will become advocates for those treatments that most help their patients, just like any other medicine.

Although prescribed DTx will likely be a powerful pillar in the therapeutic market with many products, that doesn't mean that there will be a single business model around their use or integration with other modalities. Pharma's evolving relationship with DTx serves as a good example. Over time, some pharmaceutical companies will strengthen their DTx-related capabilities with dedicated resources or departments, while others will remain focused on their traditional core business, thereby becoming potential distribution partners. For their part, DTx organizations are starting to realize that the pharmaceutical industry can be a natural ally in the development, distribution, and commercialization of DTx, and many commercialization options, alone or in a partnership, will be viable.

There is, therefore, no one-size-fits-all business model for DTx. Akili, for example, uses a market-based approach. In the United States, the company is building its own commercial distribution model that is a hybrid of key tactics from the pharmaceutical and consumer software industries, whereas in Japan it has signed a partnership with a pharmaceutical company that has deep expertise in local regulatory, marketing, and sales mechanics. Other DTx organizations may use this as inspiration . . . or not. Time will tell.

One thing is for sure: the amount of real-world data and evidence generated and collected by DTx tools far exceeds that obtained in the course of traditional drug-based therapies. This opening of the floodgates on data collection will necessarily lead to new business models, such as value-based agreements and other outcomes-based arrangements, providing greater incentives for treatments that work and less for those that do not. For now, the priority for most DTx innovators, entrepreneurs, and companies (besides obtaining regulatory clearance) is how to provide patients access to DTx. It's the responsibility of both DTx organizations as well as the larger ecosystem, including public and private payers, to crack the tough nut of moving from experimental programmatic spending to claims-based reimbursement, and, quite simply, to paying for products that are clinically proven and can enhance patients' lives, irrespective of their modality.

From Hype to Reality

There is a lot of hype in the digital health space, which is commonly accompanied by exaggerated expectations that might lead to disillusionment. DTx are not a miracle digital alternative designed to replace traditional medicine. Neither are they a marketing tactic that purports to convince you to leave your doctor and surrender into technology's arms. To rule out any temptation to conflate DTx discussions with marketing speak, we need to collectively realize the potential of these digital health tools beyond the hype. For that, DTx organizations need to invest in engaging physicians and patients early on, building trust with them over time, and having proactive communication with all stakeholders at all stages of DTx development, all the while focusing on the most critical cornerstone of generating solid clinical evidence.

Why is clinical evidence so important? As more and more startups and organizations jump on the business of health care bandwagon, the number of products, platforms, and applications that make outlandish claims and are being pushed onto physicians and patients, increases. To stand out from this crowd, DTx innovators need to arm themselves with the best tool that separates hype from reality: clinical evidence. It is the key aspect of DTx that makes all the difference and that should be the focal point of any conversation with physicians around a DTx trial, pilot, or implementation.

Technology is only a part of a solution and it cannot reinvent health care on its own. For this reason, our hope is that the experiences and insights contained in this book will serve as a how-to guide in your DTx journey and help you overcome the challenges that certainly lie ahead as you move closer to implementing your solution into existing models of care. It's time to realize the potential of DTx and improve patient outcomes at scale. *When patients need it, and you have proof it can help, it's worth the hard work to make it happen . . . and all signs are pointing to that happening in a very big way.*

NOTES

1. Mobiquity Inc., "COVID-19: Ensuring a Quality Patient Experience with the Rise of Digitisation in a Healthcare Setting"; Sham, *Accenture 2019 Digital Health Consumer Survey.*

2. Ahuja, "The Impact of Artificial Intelligence in Medicine on the Future Role of the Physician"; Goldhahn et al., "Could Artificial Intelligence Make Doctors Obsolete?"

3. Gordon, Phillips, and Beresin, "The Doctor–Patient Relationship."

ACKNOWLEDGMENTS

We are deeply grateful to Chong Yap Seng, Lien Ying Chow Professor in Medicine and Dean of the Yong Loo Lin School of Medicine, National University of Singapore (NUS Medicine). Under his visionary leadership, WisDM was established to redefine the concept of patient impact through practice-changing, multidisciplinary health care innovation. We thank Professor Chong for supporting this book project.

This book is based on the collective experience of our many contributors and experts who share our belief in the importance of raising awareness about digital therapeutics (DTx), a new class of medicine, but also about what it takes to develop, validate, and implement a new technology, especially in health care settings. We are sincerely grateful for their contributions and support. Our teams at the Institute for Digital Medicine (WisDM) at NUS Medicine, N.1 Institute for Health, and Department of Biomedical Engineering in the College of Design and Engineering at NUS have immensely contributed to the book by sharing their expertise. We would like to thank Associate Professor Christopher L. Asplund, Associate Professor B. T. Thomas Yeo, Associate Professor Jason Kai Wei Lee, and their team members for the privilege of serving as their collaborators. We would like to thank, too, Gavin Teo for helpful discussions and for his leadership and dedication toward advancing entrepreneurship and innovation in DTx.

The book is also the result of a community of patients and highly talented and committed researchers, engineers, and clinicians from the faculties and departments of NUS, NUS Medicine, and the National University Hospital in Singapore. They tirelessly push the boundaries in health care to improve patients' lives. We are fortunate to reside within one of the few ecosystems in the world that seamlessly integrates every domain that is essential to realizing health care impact at scale and the full potential of digital health—from technology and trial design to behavioral sciences and policy.

We would like to thank our amazing copyeditor, Gergana Koleva, who helped ready the manuscript, as well as everyone who reviewed the many drafts of the manuscript and generously gave us their time toward this project. We are deeply appreciative of their insights.

To Poonam Rai, Khew Si Ying, the NUS Office of Legal Affairs, and NUS Development Office, thank you for being an amazing part of our team and community. Your continuous support has been a catalyst toward everything from the successful launches of so many projects to the establishment of the Patient Impact Fund and the completion of this book.

To Sally Toh, Gladys Sim, and Michael Lim from the NUS Medicine communications team; Dr. Raja Kamal and Frank Lavin from the NUS Medicine International Council; Ron Kaufman; and the NUS Medicine finance and contracts teams. Thank you for always serving as the gateway for conveying our innovations to the broader community. Your efforts have played a vital role in bridging our work with our surrounding ecosystem. We are deeply appreciative of all of your unwavering support from the very beginning of this book project, through its development process, and to its launch.

This book would not have been possible without the enthusiasm of our agents, Nick Wallwork and Chris Newson, and our wonderful editors, Joe Rusko, Robert Brown, Alena Jones, and Adelene Jane Medrano. We are grateful for their comments and editorial feedback.

Last but not least, we would like to thank our families and close ones for their unwavering support while we embarked on this exciting and ambitious project.

AI and Its Potential Use in DTx:
A Brief Overview of Frequently Asked Questions

ALEXANDRIA MARIE REMUS, PHD

*Alexandria Marie Remus, PhD, is a DTx development specialist at the N.1
Institute for Health at the National University of Singapore.*

What Is Artificial Intelligence?

To understand the potential of applying artificial intelligence (AI) toward
digital therapeutics (DTx), one first must understand the basic concepts of
AI. AI is highly embedded in the world around us; however, misalignment
between its technical definition and daily use of the term has been confus-
ing for many aiming to enter the field. At its core, AI is a branch of computer science defined as the simulation of human intelligence in machines,
computers, or robots. In this sense, its application centers on programming
machines to think and act like humans (or sometimes animals) by "teach-
ing" them to learn, recognize, understand, respond, decide, and solve
problems on their own.

AI is being applied to many different industries, including finance,
education, transportation, health care, retail, logistics, and sports. To
understand the true potential application of AI, however, one must also be
aware of the different types and subsets of the field. A general schematic
representation of the complexity of AI according to its "strength" and the
function for which it is being deployed is depicted in figure A.1. In this
common understanding, the internal hierarchy of this field is determined
along two main branches, or types: capability (Type 1) and functionality
(Type 2). These two branches are further broken down into subcategories.

Type 1: Capability of AI

Type 1 classifies AI according to its capabilities and encompasses three
categories: artificial narrow intelligence (ANI), artificial general intelligence (AGI), and artificial super intelligence (ASI). ANI, also referred to as
weak AI, describes AI that powers a machine to perform a particular task
but does not enable the machine to have decision-making capacity, and the

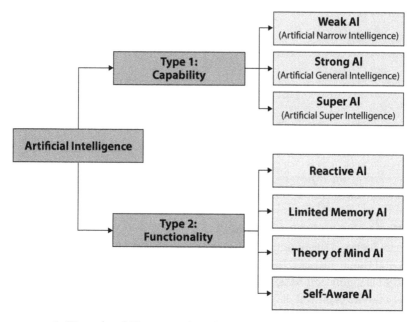

FIGURE A.1. Hierarchy of AI. Source: Adapted by permission from Springer Nature: Zelinka et al., "Artificial Intelligence in Astrophysics," 3

machine will never "pass" as a human in any other task or function outside this predefined capacity. AGI, also referred to as *strong AI*, describes AI that programs machines with the ability to learn and apply their intelligence to solve any problem and performs on par with humans. ASI, also known as *super AI*, describes AI in which machines are programmed to evolve and eventually become more intelligent than humans. These three categories of AI are described in more detail below.

WEAK AI

AI technologies that are commercialized or used in research today largely fall within the category of weak AI. Weak AI is widely leveraged in commercial applications, science, business, and health care. Its most common use is in programming machines to recognize commands and return searchable information or to detect patterns in data and classify new data accordingly. Virtual assistants such as Apple's Siri, Amazon's Alexa, and Microsoft's Cortana are good examples of this. These voice-activated devices "listen" for what they are "taught" to recognize, classify those cues, and then produce a more or less accurate response. For instance, when you ask Alexa to "play Rage Against the Machine on Spotify," the voice assistant is programmed to understand key words and phrases such as "play," "rage against the machine," and "Spotify," and will respond by playing Rage Against the Machine over the speaker. Chatbots that are often available on a business or a hospital website that are used to direct customers' inquiries run on the same principle, although their input format may be not voice but text instead. Other applications of weak AI use computers to process big data and convert them into practical bites of information by detecting patterns and making predictions; use cases include medical diagnoses, personalized song recommendations, purchase recommendations, and even email spam filters. In summary, weak AI machines do what they are told to do but do not "comprehend" the meaning of what they are asked to do or the results they produce and cannot perform outside of predefined tasks.

While the majority of these applications are deemed as positive and beneficial, since they enhance our experiences as citizens, consumers, and patients, weak AI does not come without risks. For example, systems that incorporate weak AI may fail unintentionally. Examples include disruptions in power supply or chaotic driving by autonomous vehicles. A weak AI system can also be programmed to do something good or beneficial but respond with a destructive method for achieving that goal. An example of this can be a self-driving car that is programmed to send a passenger home as quickly as possible but accomplishes this task by speeding through red lights. Because of these inherent risks of current AI architectures, integrating AI capabilities to perform any new task should be meticulously planned, tested, and evaluated.

STRONG AI

The next evolutionary stage of AI is the category of strong AI. Strong AI could endow machines with human-level intelligence but currently only exists in theory. This category of AI describes the hypothetical intelligence of a computer program that has the capacity to undertake any intellectual task a human can, such as reasoning, solving puzzles, making judgements, planning, learning, and communicating, as well as possessing consciousness, objective thoughts, self-awareness, and sentience. In contrast to weak AI, strong AI does not follow specific cues or commands to respond but instead processes the data with grouping and association rules to generate an independent and unpredictable response. What this means in practice is that there isn't a set of predefined responses the machine can choose from and reply with, which is essentially what Alexa and its peers do. Instead, it produces a novel or unpredictable result, similar to how we might expect a human to respond when asked a question.

While AGI is currently hypothetical, a recent survey of AI experts predicted its emergence by 2060.[1] Although this date is debated, with the rapid development of AI, it is reasonable to believe that applications of strong AI might appear within our lifetime or by century's end. Developments behind GPT (the "engine" of ChatGPT and Bing) are examples of significant steps toward AGI.

SUPER AI

The third category of AI is super AI. This is the kind of AI that most people think of when they talk about robots taking over the world—a common plotline in science fiction movies and books. In these fictional scenarios, AI surpasses human intelligence and ability. Again, super AI is purely speculative at this point and will most likely remain an element of science fiction for the foreseeable future.

Type 2: Functionality of AI

Type 2 classifies AI according to its functionalities and has four categories: reactive AI, limited memory AI, theory of mind AI, and self-aware AI. While this grouping is independent from the grouping based on capabilities of AI, the functionalities have similar underlying logic and applications. These four categories of AI are described in more detail below.

REACTIVE AI

Reactive AI, as the name suggests, has the functionality to "react" to a given situation and context by doing exactly what it has been programmed to do. This type of AI cannot form memories or use past experiences to make decisions. As a result, it does not learn and evolve and is therefore the most basic type of AI. The most well-known example of reactive AI is the supercomputer Deep Blue created by IBM that was programmed to play chess and challenge Garry Kasparov, the world chess champion, in 1996 and 1997.[2]

LIMITED MEMORY AI

The functionality of limited memory AI is what the term implies—a machine that has the capability to retain some information that it has learned or observed and to use it in conjunction with preprogrammed data. With this functionality, machines can observe the environment, detect patterns or changes, and respond accordingly. They do so by applying previous training on data from big datasets that are stored in the machine's memory as a reference model. These models can improve over time, unlike the static reactive AI, because they incorporate machine-learning and deep-learning models, described later in this chapter. Limited memory AI is used in most AI applications today and common examples include image classification, autonomous cars, chatbots, and virtual assistants.

THEORY OF MIND AI

Theory of mind AI describes a theoretical AI functionality whereby machines have decision-making capabilities that are equivalent to human decision-making. With this functionality, machines would be able to understand and remember not just situations but also emotions and adjust their behavior just as humans do in different social interactions and contexts. While researchers and scientists are making tremendous leaps in developing theory of mind AI, we are still some time away from seeing it in practice. There are, however, two well-known sociable robots, Kismet, developed by Dr. Cynthia Breazeal from Massachusetts Institute of Technology in the late 1990s, and Sophia, developed by Hanson Robotics in 2016, that have been developed using elements of theory of mind AI.

SELF-AWARE AI

Like theory of mind AI, self-aware AI currently only exists in theory and is imagined as an extension of theory of mind AI. Self-aware AI machines would not only be able to recognize and replicate human actions but also think for themselves, form their own desires, and understand their own feelings. This would be the most complex type of AI and—like super AI—at present exists only in the realm of science fiction. It is unknown if and when humans will be capable of developing machines with self-aware AI functionalities.

Subsets of AI

Now that we have a brief and general understanding of the two types of AI and their subcategories, let's have a look at the different subsets of AI in order to complete our picture of what AI is and how it can be applied, particularly with respect to DTx. These subsets of AI are loosely categorized by the type of analytical method or algorithm used to achieve their respective AI capability and functionality. Figure A.2 illustrates how the subsets of AI relate to each other and what applications they encompass. Machine learning (ML), and its own subset, deep learning (DL), are the most common applications of AI within a health care context and have the potential to be leveraged into DTx.

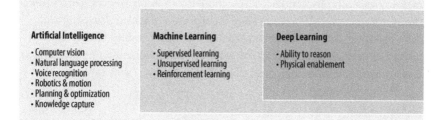

Artificial Intelligence

- Computer vision
- Natural language processing
- Voice recognition
- Robotics & motion
- Planning & optimization
- Knowledge capture

Machine Learning

- Supervised learning
- Unsupervised learning
- Reinforcement learning

Deep Learning

- Ability to reason
- Physical enablement

FIGURE A.2. Different subsets of AI. Source: Adapted from Zaleha H et al., "Intelligent Locking System Using Deep Learning for Autonomous Vehicle in Internet of Things," 568

MACHINE LEARNING

Within the overarching universe of AI, machine learning is its first and most common subset. Its foundational purpose is to "teach" computers how to learn without the necessity to be programmed for specific tasks. To achieve this, the machines are fed data and equipped with an algorithm that enables them to learn from the data and then use the insights to make predictions or other intelligent decisions. In ML models, the data input can be anything from numbers, to words, to images, to sounds, to even clicks. Most applications of AI today use machine learning in some shape or form.

Delving further, there are three approaches of machine learning, based on the expected input and output of the underlying algorithm: supervised learning, unsupervised learning, and reinforcement learning. An AI model using supervised learning relies on previously labeled data with the aim of calculating and predicting an outcome. By comparison, an AI model using unsupervised learning is trained on unlabeled data and without any guidance with the aim of discovering underlying patterns. Lastly, an AI model using reinforcement learning works by interacting with its environment, with no predefined labeled or unlabeled data, with the aim of inferring on its own a series of actions and, as the name suggests, reinforcing that learning through future iterations. The choice of one or another of these ML types depends on the problem to be solved.

DEEP LEARNING

Deep learning is one of the most rapidly developing subsets of machine learning and AI today. It describes a machine's capability to mimic the workings of the human brain and perform human-like tasks without human input. This subset of machine learning is based on a neural network model, which is a network of algorithms that attempt to replicate the perception and thought process of the human brain. A simplified neural network has three main components: (1) an input layer, where data enter the network; (2) one or more hidden, or computational, layers, where at least one algorithm processes the input data by applying learnable parameters; and (3) an output layer, where the conclusions of the model, which might take the form of predictions or diagnoses, emerge. More complex neural network models, known as deep neural networks, are comprised of many layers that interact to analyze the data and shape the final output. Generally, deep learning is the leading AI approach used in autonomous vehicles and speech recognition.

What Are Examples of Current Applications of AI in Health Care?
Current uses of AI in health care settings range from supporting personnel with day-to-day tasks, optimizing administrative workflow, and improving image analysis for diagnostics to streamlining remote patient monitoring. A few of these applications and some selected examples are detailed below.

Augmenting Diagnostics
One of the most widely used AI applications in clinical settings is diagnostics, where they are deployed to sift through electronic health record data or medical scans and discard instances in which there are no signs of disease, as well as provide further detail in cases where there may be a basis for concern. In doing so, such applications both save time for busy clinicians and reduce human error that may occur by inadvertently overlooking problematic cases. In other scenarios, ML and DL algorithms are leveraged to analyze patient clinical data—such as vital signs, symptoms, images, and other test results—with the aim of predicting probable diagnoses and outcomes. This is made possible by having previously trained the algorithms to analyze patterns in large patient datasets and to predict susceptibility to developing specific diseases based on those patterns, some of which may be too subtle for clinicians to recognize. Another application of AI in the context of diagnostics involves training algorithms to recognize anomalies—such as tumors in biopsies and various imaging modalities. In fact, a recent review identified these AI technologies to have similar or better accuracy than trained clinicians in detecting disease from medical images.[3] Some examples of AI platforms for augmenting diagnostics include PathAI (https://www.pathai.com), Buoy Health (https://www.buoyhealth .com), and BEHOLD.AI (https://behold.ai).

Augmenting Drug Discovery and Development

The traditional research and development process requires thousands of human hours and billions of dollars to develop a drug candidate, test it in clinical trials, and potentially receive a regulatory approval. Yet only a small percentage of new drugs are successfully validated and brought to market. To compress the time it takes to go through these R&D stages, AI is increasingly being used to screen large compound libraries, predict which potential compounds are likely to be effective for a certain condition, and direct a small subset of selected compounds for subsequent experimental testing. This approach results in saved time and money as compared to experimentally testing the whole compound library. Another common AI application in the context of drug development is automating labor-intensive and repetitive tasks, such as image analysis, which also leads to a reduction in human hours spent. Yet another application is using AI algorithms to screen large drug libraries to identify drugs that may be safely repurposed for treating additional indications than those for which they were originally developed. In fact, many labs globally harnessed this AI approach during the emergence of the COVID-19 pandemic to identify possible therapies while vaccine development was being pursued in parallel. Some examples of existing AI applications for augmenting drug discovery and development include IDentif.AI,[4] BioXcel Therapeutics (https://www.bioxceltherapeutics.com), Engine Biosciences (https://enginebio.com), and BenevolentAI (https://www.benevolent.com).

What Is the Potential for AI in DTx?

As discussed throughout the book, DTx platforms are on a trajectory to transform patient care. As a reminder, the Digital Therapeutics Alliance defines DTx platforms as technologies that deliver evidence-based, clinically validated therapeutic interventions, driven by validated software programs, to prevent, manage, or treat medical conditions. DTx clinical trials and their eventual deployment can generate massive volumes of data in real time at unprecedented accuracy and frequency—a perfect match for AI technologies. While we only highlighted a few current applications of AI in health care, we hope it is evident that AI has the potential to take DTx and patient care to the next level.

One of the most promising applications of the union of AI with DTx is the potential to move health care away from one-size-fits-all approaches to delivering more individualized, patient-centric interventions. DTx offer the ability to remotely collect a large amount of user data over a number of time points. These large datasets can provide deep insights into longitudinal trends and acute changes for a user, which are opportunistic for ML and DL models. Such algorithms can then be trained and harnessed to deliver personalized interventional care for users. An application of a personalized preventative intervention may involve a DTx that promotes behavioral changes that can decrease a patient's risk for developing a disease, such as the transition from a prehypertensive to hypertensive stage by promoting an increase in physical activity. Such a DTx may monitor a prehypertensive person's activity levels and use ML algorithms to identify periods of low activity to then send personalized reminders to encourage physical activity or reward the user when they perform physical activity. The resulting behavioral change of increased activity may prevent this individual from progression toward more severe stages of hypertension and may even remove them from the prehypertensive stage.

In a similar DTx that does not harness AI, all users may be subject to the same preventative intervention at the same time points regardless of their own activity levels. While a number of users may still benefit from such DTx intervention, the treatment may be suboptimal, impact compliance, and may not benefit the majority of users. Multiple other examples can be found throughout the book. Overall, the incorporation of AI in DTx solutions has the potential to deliver more personalized care to large populations without the need for a large number of specialized health care providers required to deliver such care, which in turn may improve outcomes.

What Are Some Data and Regulatory Challenges Posed by AI in DTx?

While the potential for AI-driven DTx solutions seems undeniable, there are also challenges to overcome and risks that must be assessed during the course of development as well as implementation. For example, most often AI algorithms require large amounts of data to be trained on. This requires access to mass user data in early development before an AI-driven DTx may be proven effective and beneficial. This mass collection and storage of patient data also requires AI-driven DTx solutions to implement stringent privacy and security measures to prevent data leaks. Developers also need to be aware of bias incorporated into the implemented AI algorithm if it is not trained on a diverse patient sample and must consider the safety of deploying such algorithms in a diverse sample.

Another challenge is that the AI-driven DTx technologies must still undergo the regulatory approval process. Unlike traditional therapeutics that involve the intake of drugs, the substantial amounts of data collected by an AI-enabled DTx make it possible for the underlying algorithms to improve and evolve over time. Thus, AI-DTx version 1.0 can become AI-DTx version 1.1, which can then become AI-DTx version 1.2, and so on. This potential for technological evolution raises the question of what happens if AI-DTx 1.0 gains regulatory approval but is soon after improved and upgraded—will the approval remain valid for AI-DTx 1.1 and subsequent software updates? As this field expands, the momentum for developing frameworks and guidelines for DTx that incorporate AI is continuously growing.

Signaling its readiness for this new phase, in January 2021 the US Food and Drug Administration released a plan for establishing a regulatory approach for evaluating and improving evolving AI and ML algorithms as well as advancing real-world performance pilots to provide clarity on what a real-world evidence program would look like for AI- and ML-based software as a medical device (SaMD). Similarly, in October 2021 Singapore's Ministry of Health (MOH), Health & Sciences Authority, and Integrated Health Information Systems codeveloped the MOH Artificial Intelligence in Healthcare Guidelines for both developers and implementors of AI tools in health care based in Singapore.

This is an important step in the right direction. Additional contributions to this arena from the community of international regulatory bodies will serve as an important collaborative foundation, as AI technology is also evolving during this period. Additionally, the development and adoption of established regulatory frameworks may be among the primary catalysts that rapidly advance the field.

What Is the Future of AI in DTx?

DTx have a yet-to-be-fully-tapped potential to deliver evidence-based treatment interventions to patients across many conditions in a uniquely efficient way. Its combination with AI offers insights and interventional opportunities that traditional and other digitalized therapies do not. As the field continues to grow and specific regulatory frameworks emerge, it is expected that AI-powered DTx will transform the conceptualization and delivery of health care. These opportunities to improve patient care and outcomes are endless and exciting.

NOTES

1. Dilmegani, "When Will Singularity Happen? 995 Experts' Opinions on AGI."

2. Goodrich, "How IBM's Deep Blue Beat World Champion Chess Player Garry Kasparov."

3. Liu et al., "A Comparison of Deep Learning Performance against Health-Care Professionals in Detecting Diseases from Medical Imaging."

4. Blasiak et al., "IDentif.AI: Rapidly Optimizing Combination Therapy Design against Severe Acute Respiratory Syndrome Coronavirus 2 (SARS-CoV-2) with Digital Drug Development."

How to Translate Evidence-Based Theories to the Design of
Digitally Delivered Mental Health Interventions

*This appendix was coauthored with Dr. Geck Hong Yeo, research fellow
at the N.1 Institute for Health (N.1), and Matt Oon, CEO and founder of
Acceset, a Singapore-based social enterprise. Acceset aims to transform
the management of mental health care through an anonymous text-based
therapy involving trained volunteers overseen by licensed therapists and
psychiatrists. The teams at WisDM and N.1 have been working with Acceset
to develop prospective protocols to validate, through qualitative and quantitative
research, the use of its technology to provide emotional support to Singaporean
youths struggling with anxiety and/or depression.*

In our experience working with startups involved in digital health (DH)
development, we have found that many tend to build their solutions based
on their own experiences and applied frameworks. The theoretical resources
tend to be overlooked or viewed as not being directly applicable enough to
the solution being developed and/or the condition being addressed.
Importantly, evidence-based theoretical frameworks (EBTFs) can guide
decisions on which variables to investigate and which features to include in
the solution.

Consider the story of Siam (a pseudonym), a patient battling depression.

*There is a constant inner voice that amplifies a sense of anxiety or a sense of
worthlessness and calibrating this requires a very intentional and intensive
process with the therapist, whom I'm already seeing once a week for two hours.
It is not always easy to get a consultation slot and these sessions are not the
most affordable . . . but you know that you need them to learn to dissociate
from thoughts that prevent one from feeling good about oneself—to deal with
the shame, fear and constant judgment. . . . Sometimes you feel lonely and you
have a lot of negative thoughts and feelings that eat away your worth as a
person. How one views the world, one's outlook of life, is often a mirror image
of their internal state of mind. I can see myself in the mirror and believe that*

I am not worthy. Then this can influence the outlook I have on life in general and events that occur in my life. Your family, friends, and most people in the society don't understand what you are going through, nor respect the fact that you need your space to heal. This has made recovery a truly difficult process, as I cannot control how others view me and how supportive they would be to the things I do for my own mental wellness.   —Siam, 32 years old

Siam's story is particularly insightful. It underlines the difficulties he, his family, and his doctor face in managing his disease, as well as the challenges we face as a society in aiding people suffering from depression. Like those suffering from any mental illness, they continue to endure significant stigma even today, including general social distancing stigma (being perceived as dangerous and unpredictable, as someone best avoided) and being seen as having a personal weakness, or being "weak not sick."[1]

The way society views mental health needs to change. For Siam and many others, the priority is to recognize that being depressed does not imply being "weak." Doing so will assist and empower him to better comprehend his condition and realize that he might need help. This is precisely where DTx technology can be successfully leveraged to facilitate access to mental health literacy, resources, and support in a user-centric and anonymous format. DTx may also offer the possibility to engage persons suffering from depression beyond therapist consultations. For example, it can help Siam manage his symptoms with personalized cognitive and physical exercises as well as monitor his progress. If DTx platforms have the potential to help individuals with a mental health condition, they should be designed in a way that can effect meaningful change to these individuals, including long-term behavior modification. To do so, DTx needs to rest on solid scaffolding that bridges theoretical and clinically driven underpinnings.

Interventions can be based on varying segments along the theoretical to clinical/user continuum. Where applicable, a theoretical basis for intervention design—such as the exploration of mattering-based digital peer support—could indeed be important when designing mental health solutions. This foundation provides a set of principles guiding how different aspects or elements of social phenomena relate to each other and can direct our use of DTx. A theory is defined as a set of principles governing how different aspects or elements of social phenomena relate to each other.[2] As an organizing framework, it accounts for what is known, explains the current state, and predicts future phenomena. These principles of a theory are generated from scientific methods and grounded in empirical evidence.

To emphasize the importance of evidence in supporting eventual DTx deployment, the development and evaluation of DTx platforms informed by principles that are generated from scientific methods and grounded in empirical evidence may ultimately be more clinically effective than those that aren't. For these reasons, we recommend that researchers, practitioners, and budding DTx entrepreneurs build teams with experience in validating evidence-based theories and frameworks for the purpose of developing high-quality DTx solutions. Here Dr. Geck Hong Yeo and Matt Oon share some of their experiences translating theoretical and empirical research into real-world applications of designing DTx for addressing mental health needs.

Why Is An Evidence-Based Theoretical Framework Useful for DTx in General?

The Story behind Acceset, by Mr. Oon

I have been a caregiver to my mother, who has schizophrenia, since I was 7 years old. The responsibilities I had to take on throughout the years seeded my interest for mental health issues. In the very beginning, being her caregiver inspired me to volunteer for initiatives supporting the mental well-being of young people in Singapore. This is where I discovered my passion for innovation and driving social change. I also witnessed that physical clinics and peer networks had limitations in engendering help-seeking behavior among youth. They didn't provide sufficient protection of their identity, nor did they give them control over the medium and mode of emotional disclosure. The development of Acceset stemmed from the belief that lending a listening ear to struggling youths in Singapore was what they really needed.

Today Acceset provides anonymous text-based therapy through a digital letter-writing platform, which offers a safe space for those who want to share their concerns anonymously and receive support. We strive to make emotional support easily accessible to youths while educating them on mental health care, by leveraging technology as well as qualitative and quantitative research.

Working on Theories with Acceset, by Dr. Yeo

Specific to Acceset, a sound evidence-based framework at the conception stage would address critical questions, such as why Acceset is focusing on online peer support. What form of peer support should Acceset enable? What features of the online peer support system should Acceset include that will facilitate peer disclosure online?

It is true for Acceset, as it is for all digital health technologies, that it is critical to identify a sound, relevant, and empirically supported theoretical framework. The alternative and too common "post hoc" approach, whereby developers would design and implement the DH solution and then try to retrofit it with a relevant theoretical framework, leads to downstream issues, such as failing to include relevant or key features of DH that are needed to address the health concerns that the DH was originally intended for (or including irrelevant ones). It also presents potential cost-effectiveness concerns associated with the technology needed for the DH. The next step, therefore, is to identify an appropriate EBTF.

How Do You Determine If an Evidence-Based Theoretical Framework Is Relevant to Your Mental Health Solution?

From our experience, it is useful to consider the following five questions to help you identify a sound and relevant EBTF for your mental health solution:

1. Does the theory describe and explain the links between the outcomes that the DTx is designed to measure and intervene upon?
2. Is there information outlining the application of the theory to a mental health intervention, especially in the envisioned intervention context (e.g., features of the individuals and community, modes of intervention)?
3. Has this theory already been applied in longitudinal studies (i.e., investigating change in mental health behaviors over time) and/or translational research (i.e., examining the mechanism of change between the intervention and mental health outcomes/changes, or the steps or path in which the intervention leads to mental health outcomes/changes)?
4. Is there evidence for the application of the theory to an intervention that has demonstrated change in the expected magnitude and direction in mental health outcomes or behaviors?
5. Is there information/evidence that clearly defines the mechanism of action?

Mattering as an Evidence-Based Theory for Acceset, by Mr. Oon

For Acceset, it is the mattering theory that informed our solution. The mattering theory refers to the extent to which we make a difference to the world in which we live.[3] It resonates strongly with youths' lived experiences of anxiety and depression. For this group of individuals, it can instill a sense of significance and offers a specific positive framing for addressing mental health issues. We are therefore focused on conveying an increased sense of mattering through digital interventions that can boost the well-being of the adolescents.

Deciding on Mattering as a Potential Framework for Acceset, by Dr. Yeo
We went through the five key questions in thinking about and deciding on a theory that would be the most appropriate in the design of Acceset as a digital peer intervention in support of adolescents' mental well-being. Here is the outline of the thought processes for three of these questions:

1. *Does the theory describe and explain the links between the outcomes that the DTx is designed to measure and intervene upon?*

    Mattering is comprised of attention, importance, and reliance. Recent studies seek to understand the role of mattering in adolescents' well-being, such as being a potential "active ingredient" in interventions aimed at mitigating adolescent anxiety and depression.[4] Thus, we are investigating mattering as a relevant EBTF for developing and strengthening Acceset's solution.

    Acceset's platform underscores the building of interpersonal relationships that enhance their sense of mattering. Through the disclosure of emotionally laden experiences online with one's peers, and their peers' supportive responses, adolescents receive attention that is much needed for helping them manage how they express and regulate their emotions. This interpersonal exchange may improve their sense of importance and reliance, as adolescents feel that their needs and concerns are heard, and they can rely for support on others who share similar experiences. This may also contribute to a sense of meaning and purpose and overall well-being.

2. *Is there information outlining the application of the theory to a mental health intervention, especially in the envisioned intervention context?*

    Theory and research on mattering has been applied to understand and support adolescents' anxiety and depression, including their lived experiences comprising irrational thoughts, fear, lack of control, and feelings of insignificance.[5] Research on mattering demonstrated significant gender differences—specifically, females perceived a higher overall sense of mattering and domain-specific mattering related to family, school, and friends—with only one study documenting nongendered effects.[6] Such information is pertinent in the design of a solution as a mental health intervention.

In terms of age differences in mattering, there are also findings that hint at the relative importance of mattering to the family and peer domains for young adults and adolescents, respectively.[7]

3. *Has this theory already been applied in longitudinal studies and/or translational research?*

Research documented the steps in how mattering impacts psychological well-being. Mattering is related to one's selfhood and is distinguished from other important self domains, such as self-esteem and self-presentation. Increasing one's sense of mattering, in turn, increases self-esteem, which contributes to or supports youths' well-being.[8]

Conclusion

By translating theoretical and empirical research into the conceptualization, design, operationalization, and real-world application of DTx, DTx entrepreneurs can efficiently and effectively leverage technology to improve the mental health of young people and of society as a whole. We therefore recommend exploring the role of evidence-based theoretical frameworks as a guide to help pinpoint features to incorporate in a given solution as well as clinical outcomes to assess by way of providing evidence for the effectiveness of that solution. Therefore, in the design stage, we encourage you to think about these next questions as key pointers in applying an EBTF in the design of your solution:

1. What does the evidence-based theory specify to be an effective component or "active ingredient" of the intervention?
2. What are the key characteristics or features of the solution that function as the intervention for the gap you are addressing?
3. How do these defining characteristics of the solution map onto the effective components or active ingredients specified by the theory?
4. What are the underlying operating principles, assumptions, and relations between the effective components or active ingredients outlined by the evidence-based theory?
5. How does this evidence-based theory explain how different effective components or active ingredients of your solution interact with one another in producing an effect to function as an intervention?

The application of an evidence-based theoretical framework should not be limited to the conceptualization of your solution but also considered for its operationalization, as we discuss in Part III of the book.

NOTES

1. Subramaniam et al., "Stigma towards People with Mental Disorders and Its Components."

2. Moller et al., "Applying and Advancing Behavior Change Theories and Techniques in the Context of a Digital Health Revolution."

3. Elliott, Kao, and Grant, "Mattering: Empirical Validation of a Social-Psychological Concept."

4. Marshall and Tilton-Weaver, "Adolescents' Perceived Mattering to Parents and Friends"; Flett et al., "Academic Buoyancy and Mattering as Resilience Factors in Chinese Adolescents."

5. Flett, Burdo, and Nepon, "Mattering, Insecure Attachment, Rumination, and Self-Criticism in Distress among University Students"; Matera, Bosco, and Meringolo, "Perceived Mattering to Family and Friends, Self-Esteem, and Well-Being."

6. Marshall and Tilton-Weaver, "Adolescents' Perceived Mattering to Parents and Friends"; Elliott, Colangelo, and Gelles, "Mattering and Suicide Ideation"; Marshall, "Do I Matter?"; Dixon, Scheidegger, and McWhirter, "The Adolescent Mattering Experience."

7. Dixon, Scheidegger, and McWhirter, "The Adolescent Mattering Experience"; Finkel and Baumeister, *Advanced Social Psychology: The State of the Science*.

8. Flett and Nepon, "Mattering versus Self-Esteem in University Students: Associations with Regulatory Focus, Social Feedback, and Psychological Distress."

Adler, Nancy E., and Ann E. K. Page, eds. *Cancer Care for the Whole Patient: Meeting Psychosocial Health Needs*. Washington, DC: National Academies Press, 2008. https://www.ncbi.nlm.nih.gov/books/NBK4015.

Ahmad, Amar S., Nick Ormiston-Smith, and Peter D. Sasieni. "Trends in the Lifetime Risk of Developing Cancer in Great Britain: Comparison of Risk for those Born from 1930 to 1960." *British Journal of Cancer* 112, no. 5 (2015): 943–47. https://doi.org/10.1038/bjc.2014.606.

Ahuja, Abhimanyu S. "The Impact of Artificial Intelligence in Medicine on the Future Role of the Physician." *PeerJ* 7 (2019): e7702. https://doi.org/10.7717/peerj.7702.

Akili Interactive. "Akili and Shionogi Announce Strategic Partnership to Develop and Commercialize Digital Therapeutics in Key Asian Markets." Press release, March 17, 2019. https://www.akiliinteractive.com/news-collection/akili-and-shionogi-announce-strategic-partnership-to-develop-and-commercialize-digital-therapeutics-in-key-asian-markets.

Akili Interactive. "Akili Announces FDA Clearance of EndeavorRx™ for Children with ADHD, the First Prescription Treatment Delivered through a Video Game." Press release, June 15, 2020. https://www.akiliinteractive.com/news-collection/akili-announces-endeavortm-attention-treatment-is-now-available-for-children-with-attention-deficit-hyperactivity-disorder-adhd-al3pw.

Alagizy, H. A., M. R. Soltan, S. S. Soliman, N. N. Hegazy, and S. F. Gohar. "Anxiety, Depression, and Perceived Stress among Breast Cancer Patients: Single Institute Experience." *Middle East Current Psychiatry* 27 (2020): 29. https://doi.org/10.1186/s43045-020-00036-x.

American Diabetes Association. "The Cost of Diabetes." March 22, 2018. https://www.diabetes.org/resources/statistics/cost-diabetes.

American Diabetes Association. "Insulin Myths and Facts." *Clinical Diabetes* 25, no. 1 (2007): 39–40. https://doi.org/10.2337/diaclin.25.1.39.

American Psychological Association. "What Is Cognitive Behavioral Therapy?" PTSD Clinical Practice Guideline. Accessed November 17, 2022. https://www.apa.org/ptsd-guideline/patients-and-families /cognitive-behavioral.pdf.

Anderson, Annick, Deborah Borfitz, and Kenneth Getz. "Global Public Attitudes about Clinical Research and Patient Experiences with Clinical Trials." *JAMA Network Open* 1, no. 6 (2018): e182969. https://doi.org/10 .1001/jamanetworkopen.2018.2969.

Angelis, Aris, David Tordrup, and Panos Kanavos. "Socio-Economic Burden of Rare Diseases: A Systematic Review of Cost of Illness Evidence." *Health Policy* 119, no. 7 (2015): 964–79. https://doi.org/10.1016/j.healthpol.2014 .12.016.

Anthony, Scott D., Mark W. Johnson, Joseph V. Sinfield, and Elizabeth J. Altman. *The Innovator's Guide to Growth: Putting Disruptive Innovation to Work*. Boston: Harvard Business Review Press, 2008.

Aref-Adib, Golnar, Tayla McCloud, Jamie Ross, Puffin O'Hanlon, Victoria Appleton, Sarah Rowe, Elizabeth Murray, Sonia Johnson, and Fiona Lobban. "Factors Affecting Implementation of Digital Health Interventions for People with Psychosis or Bipolar Disorder, and their Family and Friends: A Systematic Review." *Lancet Psychiatry* 6, no. 3 (2019): 257–66. https://doi.org/10.1016/S2215-0366(18)30302-X.

Arnhold, Madlen, Mandy Quade, and Wilhelm Kirch, "Mobile Applications for Diabetics: A Systematic Review and Expert-Based Usability Evaluation Considering the Special Requirements of Diabetes Patients Aged 50 Years or Older." *Journal of Medical Internet Research* 16, no. 4 (2014): e104. https://doi.org/10.2196/JMIR.2968.

Barclay, Laurie. "Exubera Approved Despite Initial Lung Function Concerns." *Medscape Medical News*, February 9, 2006. https://www.medscape .com/viewarticle/523294.

Barker, Pierre M., Amy Reid, and Marie W. Schall. "A Framework for Scaling Up Health Interventions: Lessons from Large-Scale Improvement Initiatives in Africa." *Implementation Science* 11, no. 1 (2015): 1–11. https://doi.org/10.1186/s13012-016-0374-x.

Beede, Emma, Elizabeth Baylor, Fred Hersch, Anna Iurchenko, Lauren Wilcox, Paisan Ruamviboonsuk, and Laura M. Vardoulakis. "A Human-Centered Evaluation of a Deep Learning System Deployed in Clinics for the Detection of Diabetic Retinopathy." In *Proceedings of the 2020 CHI Conference on Human Factors in Computing Systems*, (New York: Association

for Computing Machinery, 2020), 1–12. https://doi.org/10.1145/3313831
.3376718.

Belluck, Pam, and Rebecca Robbins. "FDA Approves Alzheimer's Drug
Despite Fierce Debate Over Whether It Works." *New York Times*, June 7,
2021. https://www.nytimes.com/2021/06/07/health/aduhelm-fda
-alzheimers-drug.html.

Bestsennyy, Oleg, Greg Gilbert, Alex Harris, and Jennifer Rost. "Telehealth: A Quarter-Trillion-Dollar Post-COVID-19 Reality?" McKinsey &
Company, July 9, 2021. https://www.mckinsey.com/industries/healthcare
-systems-and-services/our-insights/telehealth-a-quarter-trillion-dollar
-post-covid-19-reality.

Blasiak, Agata, Jhin Jieh Lim, Shirley Gek Kheng Seah, Theodore Kee,
Alexandria Remus, De Hoe Chye, Pui San Wong, et al. "IDentif.AI:
Rapidly Optimizing Combination Therapy Design against Severe Acute
Respiratory Syndrome Coronavirus 2 (SARS-CoV-2) with Digital Drug
Development." *Bioengineering & Translational Medicine* 6, no. 1 (2021):
e10196. https://doi.org/10.1002/btm2.10196.

Blue Note Therapeutics. "Cancer-Related Distress." Accessed July 4, 2021.
https://bluenotetherapeutics.com/why.

Boersma, Peter, Lindsey I. Black, and Brian W. Ward. "Prevalence of Multiple
Chronic Conditions among US Adults, 2018." *Preventing Chronic Disease* 17 (2020). https://doi.org//10.5888/pcd17.200130.

Bombard, Yvonne, G. Ross Baker, Elaina Orlando, Carol Fancott, Pooja
Bhatia, Selina Casalino, Kanecy Onate, Jean-Louis Denis, and Marie-
Pascale Pomey. "Engaging Patients to Improve Quality of Care: A Systematic Review." *Implementation Science* 13 (2018): 98. https://doi.org/10
.1186/s13012-018-0784-z.

Braithwaite, Jeffrey, Peter D. Hibbert, Adam Jaffe, Les White, Christopher T. Cowell, Mark F. Harris, William B. Runciman, et al. "Quality of
Health Care for Children in Australia, 2012–2013." *JAMA* 319, no. 11
(2018): 1113–24. https://doi.org/10.1001/jama.2018.0162.

Bridge Point Capital. "Advancement of Digital Therapeutics Leads to a
Huge Market with Enormous Potential." Accessed October 15, 2020.
https://www.bridgepoint.capital/post/advancement-of-digital
-therapeutics-leads-to-a-huge-market-with-enormous-potential.

Brown, Marie T., and Jennifer K. Bussell. "Medication Adherence: WHO
Cares?" *Mayo Clinic Proceedings* 86, no. 4, (2011): 304–14. https://doi.org
/10.4065/mcp.2010.0575.

Buttorff, Christine, Teague Ruder, and Melissa Bauman. *Multiple Chronic Conditions in the United States*. Vol. 10. Santa Monica, CA: Rand, 2017. https://www.rand.org/pubs/tools/TL221.html.

Byrne, Jane. "DIA 2021 Set to Shed Some Light on Decentralized Trials Process, Accelerated Approval Pathways." *BioPharma-Reporter*, June 16, 2021. https://www.biopharma-reporter.com/Article/2021/06/16/DIA -2021-set-to-shed-some-light-on-decentralized-trials-process-accelerated -approval-pathways.

Califf, Robert M., Deborah A. Zarin, Judith M. Kramer, Rachel E. Sherman, Laura H. Aberle, and Asba Tasneem. "Characteristics of Clinical Trials Registered in ClinicalTrials.gov, 2007–2010." *JAMA* 307, no. 17 (2012): 1838–47. https://doi.org/10.1001/jama.2012.3424.

CB Insights. "The Top 12 Reasons Startups Fail." August 3, 2021. https:// www.cbinsights.com/research/startup-failure-reasons-top.

Centers for Diseases Control and Prevention. "Health and Economic Costs of Chronic Diseases." Accessed November 17, 2022. https://www.cdc.gov /chronicdisease/about/costs.

Centers for Disease Control and Prevention. *National Diabetes Statistics Report 2020: Estimates of Diabetes and Its Burden in the United States*. Atlanta, GA: Centers for Disease Control and Prevention, US Depart-ment of Health and Human Services, 2020. https://www.cdc.gov /diabetes/pdfs/data/statistics/national-diabetes-statistics-report.pdf.

Centers for Disease Control and Prevention. "Workplace Health Promotion: Depression Evaluation Measures." Accessed November 17, 2022. https:// www.cdc.gov/workplacehealthpromotion/health-strategies/depression /evaluation-measures/index.html.

Centro Criptológico Nacional [National Cryptologic Center]. "Requisitos de seguridad para aplicaciones de cibersalud [Security Requirements for eHealth Applications]." September 7, 2020. https://www.ccn-cert.cni.es /comunicacion-eventos/comunicados-ccn-cert/10471-requisitos-de -seguridad-para-aplicaciones-de-cibersalud.html.

Chan, Eugene Y., and Najam U. Saqib. "Privacy Concerns Can Explain Unwillingness to Download and Use Contact Tracing Apps when COVID-19 Concerns Are High." *Computers in Human Behavior* 119 (June 2021): 106718. https://doi.org/10.1016/j.chb.2021.106718.

Chen, Sharon, and Sterling Wong. "Singapore Beats Hong Kong in Health Efficiency: Southeast Asia." *Bloomberg*, September 17, 2014. https://www .bloomberg.com/news/articles/2014-09-18/singapore-beats-hong-kong -in-health-efficiency-southeast-asia.

Christensen, Clayton M., Taddy Hall, Karen Dillon, and David S. Duncan. "Know Your Customers' 'Jobs to be Done.'" *Harvard Business Review* 94, no. 9 (2016): 54–62. https://hbr.org/2016/09/know-your-customers-jobs-to-be-done.

Choi, Mi Joo, Hana Kim, Hyun-Wook Nah, and Dong-Wha Kang, "Digital Therapeutics: Emerging New Therapy for Neurologic Deficits after Stroke." *Journal of Stroke* 21, no. 3 (2019): 242–58. https://doi.org/10.5853/jos.2019.01963.

Chudasama, Rajesh K., A. M. Kadri, Apurva Ratnu, Mahima Jain, and Chandrakant P. Kamariya. "Magnitude of Gestational Diabetes Mellitus, Its Influencing Factors, and Diagnostic Accuracy of Capillary Blood Testing for Its Detection at a Tertiary Care Centre, Rajkot, Gujarat." *Indian Journal of Community Medicine* 44, no. 2 (2019): 142–46. https://pubmed.ncbi.nlm.nih.gov/31333293.

Clement, Innocent, Andreas Lorenz, Bernhard Ulm, Anne Plidschun, and Stephan Huber. "Implementing Systematically Collected User Feedback to Increase User Retention in a Mobile App for Self-Management of Low Back Pain: Retrospective Cohort Study." *JMIR mHealth and uHealth* 6, no. 6 (2018): e10422. https://doi.org/10.2196/10422.

Clinical Trials Transformation Initiative (CTTI). *CTTI Recommendations: Decentralized Clinical Trials.* Durham, NC: CTTI, September 2018. https://ctti-clinicaltrials.org/wp-content/uploads/2021/06/CTTI_DCT_Recs.pdf.

Clinical Trials Transformation Initiative (CTTI). *Developing Novel Endpoints Generated by Digital Health Technology for Use in Clinical Trials.* Durham, NC: CTTI, April 2022. https://ctti-clinicaltrials.org/wp-content/uploads/2022/03/CTTI-Digital-Health-Trials-Novel-Endpoint-Acceptance-Recommendations.pdf.

Clinical Trials Transformation Initiative (CTTI). *Digital Health Trials: Recommendations for Delivering an Investigational Product.* Durham, NC: CTTI, July 8, 2021. https://ctti-clinicaltrials.org/wp-content/uploads/2021/07/CTTI_Delivering_an_Investigational_Product_Recommendations.pdf.

Coravos, Andrea, Jennifer C. Goldsack, Daniel R. Karlin, Camille Nebeker, Eric Perakslis, Noah Zimmerman, and M. Kelley Erb. "Digital Medicine: A Primer on Measurement." *Digital Biomarkers* 3, no. 2 (2019): 31–71. https://doi.org/10.1159/000500413.

Cosgrove, Lisa, Ioana Alina Cristea, Allen F. Shaughnessy, Barbara Mintzes, and Florian Naudet. "Digital Aripiprazole or Digital Evergreening?

A Systematic Review of the Evidence and Its Dissemination in the Scientific Literature and in the Media." *BMJ Evidence-Based Medicine* 24, no. 6 (2019): 231–38. https://doi.org/10.1136/bmjebm-2019-111204.

Darden, Michael, Colin A. Espie, Jenna R. Carl, Alasdair L. Henry, Jennifer C. Kanady, Andrew D. Krystal, Christopher B. Miller. "Cost-Effectiveness of Digital Cognitive Behavioral Therapy (*Sleepio*) for Insomnia: A Markov Simulation Model in the United States." *Sleep* 44, no. 4 (2021): zsaa223. https://doi.org/10.1093/sleep/zsaa223.

David, Daniel, Ioana Cristea, and Stefan G. Hofmann. "Why Cognitive Behavioral Therapy Is the Current Gold Standard of Psychotherapy." *Frontiers in Psychiatry* 9 (2018): 4. https://doi.org/10.3389/fpsyt.2018.00004.

Davidai, Shai, Thomas Gilovich, and Lee D. Ross. "The Meaning of Default Options for Potential Organ Donors." *Proceedings of the National Academy of Sciences* 109, no. 38 (2012): 15201–5. https://doi.org/10.1073/pnas.1211695109.

Davis, Christian, Emily Burgen, and Guoqing J. Chen. "Out-of-Pocket Costs for Patients with Type 2 Diabetes Mellitus." *Diabetes* 67, supplement 1 (2018): 2324-PUB. https://doi.org/10.2337/db18-2324-PUB.

Dean Foods and Livongo Health. *Livongo Drives 1.4x ROI in Year 1 for Dean Foods: Enrollment and Activation Best Practices Accelerate Outcomes* (case study). Dallas, TX: Dean Foods and Livongo Health, 2021. https://content.livongo.com/DEANFOODS/CaseStudy.pdf.

Derksen, Frans, Jozien Bensing, and Antoine Lagro-Janssen. "Effectiveness of Empathy in General Practice: A Systematic Review." *British Journal of General Practice* 63, no. 606 (2013): e76-e84. https://doi.org/10.3399/bjgp13X660814.

Dilmegani, Cem. "When Will Singularity Happen? 995 Experts' Opinions on AGI." AI Multiple, August 3, 2017. https://research.aimultiple.com/artificial-general-intelligence-singularity-timing.

Digital Therapeutics Alliance. *Digital Health Industry Categorization.* Arlington, VA: Digital Therapeutics Alliance, November 2019. https://dtxalliance.org/wp-content/uploads/2019/11/DTA_Digital-Industry-Categorization_Nov19.pdf.

Digital Therapeutics Alliance. *Digital Therapeutics Definition and Core Principles.* Arlington, VA: Digital Therapeutics Alliance, November 2019. https://dtxalliance.org/wp-content/uploads/2019/11/DTA_DTx-Definition-and-Core-Principles.pdf.

Digital Therapeutics Alliance. "DTx by Country." Accessed April 5, 2022. https://dtxalliance.org/understanding-dtx/dtx-by-country.

Digital Therapeutics Alliance. *DTx Product Best Practices*. Arlington, VA: Digital Therapeutics Alliance, November 2019. https://dtxalliance.org /wp-content/uploads/2019/11/DTA_DTx-Product-Best-Practices_11.11 .19.pdf.

Digital Therapeutics Alliance. "DTx Product Profile: BlueStar." Accessed November 17, 2022. https://dtxalliance.org/productbluestar.

Digital Therapeutics Alliance. *Ensuring Appropriate Quality, Access, and Utilization of Digital Therapeutics*. Arlington, VA: Digital Therapeutics Alliance, April 2020. https://dtxalliance.org/wp-content/uploads/2020 /04/DTx_Quality_Access_Utilization_Worksheet.pdf.

Digital Therapeutics Alliance. "Finding Value in Digital Therapeutics during COVID-19." March 19, 2020. https://dtxalliance.org/2020/03/19 /finding-value-in-dtx-products-during-covid-19.

Digital Therapeutics Alliance. "Understanding DTx." May 21, 2021. https://dtxalliance.org/understanding-dtx.

Dixon, Andrea L., Corey Scheidegger, J. Jeffries McWhirter. "The Adolescent Mattering Experience: Gender Variations in Perceived Mattering, Anxiety, and Depression." *Journal of Counseling & Development* 87, no. 3 (2011): 302–10. https://doi.org/10.1002/j.1556-6678.2009.tb00111.x.

Egede, Leonard E., Mulugeta Gebregziabher, Clara E. Dismuke, Cheryl P. Lynch, R. Neal Axon, Yumin Zhao, and Patrick D. Mauldin. "Medication Nonadherence in Diabetes: Longitudinal Effects on Costs and Potential Cost Savings from Improvement." *Diabetes Care* 35, no. 12 (2012): 2533–39. https://doi.org/10.2337/dc12-0572.

eHealth Stakeholder Group. *Proposed Guiding Principles for Reimbursement of Digital Health Products and Solutions*. Luxembourg: Medtech Europe. Accessed April 5, 2022. https://www.medtecheurope.org/wp-content /uploads/2019/04/30042019_eHSGSubGroupReimbursement.pdf.

Elliott, Gregory, Melissa F. Colangelo, and Richard J. Gelles. "Mattering and Suicide Ideation: Establishing and Elaborating a Relationship." *Social Psychology Quarterly* 68, no. 3 (2005): 223–38. https://doi.org/10 .1177/019027250506800303.

Elliott, Gregory, Suzanne Kao, and Ann-Marie Grant. "Mattering: Empirical Validation of a Social-Psychological Concept." *Self and Identity* 3, no. 4 (2010): 339–54. https://doi.org/10.1080/13576500444000119.

Espie, Colin A., Simon D. Kyle, Chris Williams, Jason C. Ong, Neil J. Douglas, Peter Hames, and June S. L. Brown. "A Randomized, Placebo-Controlled Trial of Online Cognitive Behavioral Therapy for Chronic Insomnia Disorder Delivered via an Automated Media-Rich Web

Application." *Sleep* 35, no. 6 (2012): 769–81. https://doi.org/10.5665/sleep.1872.

European Commission. "Internal Market, Industry, Entrepreneurship, and SMEs: Conformity Assessment." Accessed November 1, 2021. https://ec.europa.eu/growth/single-market/goods/building-blocks/conformity-assessment_en.

The European Union Medical Device Regulation, May 26, 2021. https://eumdr.com.

Farr, Christina. "Proteus Digital Health, Once Valued at $1.5 Billion, Files for Chapter 11 Bankruptcy." *CNBC*, June 16, 2020. https://www.cnbc.com/2020/06/15/proteus-digital-health-once-worth-1point5-billion-files-for-chapter-11.html.

Fiagbe, J., S. Bosoka, J. Opong, W. Takramah, W. K. Axame, R. Owusu, P. A. Parbey, M. Adjuik, E. Tarkang, and M. Kweku. "Prevalence of Controlled and Uncontrolled Diabetes Mellitus and Associated Factors of Controlled Diabetes among Diabetic Adults in the Hohoe Municipality of Ghana." *Diabetes Management* 7, no. 5 (2017): 343–54.

Federal Ministry of Health. "Driving the Digital Transformation of Germany's Healthcare System for the Good of Patients: The Act to Improve Healthcare Provision through Digitalisation and Innovation (Digital Healthcare Act—DVG)." Last updated April 22, 2020. https://www.bundesgesundheitsministerium.de/digital-healthcare-act.html.

Finkel, Eli J., and Roy F. Baumeister (eds.). *Advanced Social Psychology: The State of the Science*. Oxford: Oxford University Press, 2019.

Fitzsimmons-Craft, Ellen E., C. Barr Taylor, Andrea K. Graham, Shiri Sadeh-Sharvit, Katherine N. Balantekin, Dawn M. Eichen, Grace E. Monterubio, et al. "Effectiveness of a Digital Cognitive Behavior Therapy–Guided Self-Help Intervention for Eating Disorders in College Women: A Cluster Randomized Clinical Trial." *JAMA Network Open* 3, no. 8 (2020): e2015633. https://doi.org/10.1001/jamanetworkopen.2020.15633.

Flett, Gordon L., Ron Burdo, and Taryn Nepon. "Mattering, Insecure Attachment, Rumination, and Self-Criticism in Distress among University Students." *International Journal of Mental Health and Addiction* 19 (2020): 1300–13.

Flett, Gordon L., and Taryn Nepon. "Mattering versus Self-Esteem in University Students: Associations with Regulatory Focus, Social Feedback, and Psychological Distress." *Journal of Psychoeducational Assessment* 38, no. 6 (2020): 663–74. https://doi.org/10.1177/0734282919890786.

Flett, Gordon L., Chang Su, Liang Ma, and Lianrong Guo. "Academic Buoyancy and Mattering as Resilience Factors in Chinese Adolescents: An Analysis of Shame, Social Anxiety, and Psychological Distress." *International Journal of Child and Adolescent Resilience* 2, no. 1 (2014): 37–45. https://www.ijcar-rirea.ca/index.php/ijcar-rirea/article/view/159.

Forrester. "The Biggest Digital Health Deal of All Time: Teladoc and Livongo." *Forbes*, August 7, 2020. https://www.forbes.com/sites/forrester/2020/08 /07/the-biggest-digital-health-deal-of-all-time-teladoc-and-livongo.

Fraunhofer Institute for Algorithms and Scientific Computing SCAI. "Preventive Treatment for Alzheimer's and Parkinson's Disease." Fraunhofer-Gesellschaft, June 1, 2018. https://www.fraunhofer.de/en /press/research-news/2018/june/preventive-treatment-for-alzheimers -and-parkinsons-disease.html.

Gallagher, Paul. "GP Appointments Should Be at least 15 Minutes in Future, Leading Doctors Say." *iNews*, May 21, 2019. https://inews.co.uk /news/health/gp-appointments-15-minutes-standard-length-royal -college-293235.

Garavand, Ali, Mohammah Mohseni, Heshmatollah Asadi, Manal Etemadi, Mohammad Moradi-Joo, and Ahmad Moosavi. "Factors Influencing the Adoption of Health Information Technologies: A Systematic Review." *Electronic Physician* 8, no. 8 (2016): 2713–18. https://doi.org/10.19082/2713.

Gleason-Comstock, Julie, Alicia Streater, Allen Goodman, James Janisse, Aaron Brody, LynnMarie Mango, Rachelle Dawood, and Phillip Levy. "Willingness to Pay and Willingness to Accept in a Patient-Centered Blood Pressure Control Study." *BMC Health Services Research* 17, no. 1 (2017): 1–6. https://doi.org/10.1186/s12913-017-2451-5.

Granja, Conceição, Wouter Janssen, and Monika Alise Johansen. "Factors Determining the Success and Failure of eHealth Interventions: Systematic Review of the Literature." *Journal of Medical Internet Research* 20, no. 5 (2018): e10235. https://doi.org/10.2196/10235.

Greene, Jessica, Judith H. Hibbard, Rebecca Sacks, Valerie Overton, and Carmen D. Parrotta. "When Patient Activation Levels Change, Health Outcomes and Costs Change, Too." *Health Affairs* 34, no. 3 (2015): 431–37. https://doi.org/10.1377/hlthaff.2014.0452.

Greenhalgh, Trisha, and Chrysanthi Papoutsi. "Spreading and Scaling Up Innovation and Improvement." *BMJ* 365 (May 2019). https://doi.org/10 .1136/bmj.l2068.

Greenhalgh, Trisha, Joseph Wherton, Chrysanthi Papoutsi, Jennifer Lynch, Gemma Hughes, Susan Hinder, Nick Fahy, Rob Procter, and Sara

Shaw. "Beyond Adoption: A New Framework for Theorizing and Evaluating Nonadoption, Abandonment, and Challenges to the Scale-Up, Spread, and Sustainability of Health and Care Technologies." *Journal of Medical Internet Research* 19, no. 11 (2017): e367. https://doi.org/10.2196/jmir.8775.

Grefkes, Christian, and Gereon R. Fink. "Recovery from Stroke: Current Concepts and Future Perspectives." *Neurological Research and Practice* 2 (2020): 17. https://doi.org/10.1186/s42466-020-00060-6.

Goldhahn, Jörg, Vanessa Rampton, Branco Weiss, and Giatgen A. Spinas. "Could Artificial Intelligence Make Doctors Obsolete?" *BMJ* 363 (2018). https://doi.org/10.1136/bmj.k4563.

Gonzalez, Jeffrey S., Lauren A. McCarl, Deborah J. Wexler, Enrico Cagliero, Linda Delahanty, Tiffany D. Soper, Valerie Goldman, Robert Knauz, and Steven A. Safren. "Cognitive–Behavioral Therapy for Adherence and Depression (CBT-AD) in Type 2 Diabetes." *Journal of Cognitive Psychotherapy* 24, no. 4 (2010): 329–43. https://doi.org/10.1891/0889-8391.24.4.329.

Goodrich, Joanna. "How IBM's Deep Blue Beat World Champion Chess Player Garry Kasparov." *IEEE Spectrum*, January 25, 2021. https://spectrum.ieee.org/how-ibms-deep-blue-beat-world-champion-chess-player-garry-kasparov.

Gordon, Christopher, Margot Phillips, Eugene V. Beresin. "The Doctor–Patient Relationship." In *Massachusetts General Hospital Handbook of General Hospital Psychiatry*, 6th ed., edited by Theodore A. Stern, Gregory L. Fricchione, Ned H. Cassem, Michael Jellinek, and Jerrold F. Rosenbaum, 15–23. Philadelphia: W. B. Saunders, 2010. https://doi.org/10.1016/B978-1-4377-1927-7.00003-0.

Gottlieb, Scott. "Breaking Down Barriers between Clinical Trials and Clinical Care: Incorporating Real World Evidence into Regulatory Decision Making." Speech to the Bipartisan Policy Center. US Food and Drug Administration, January 28, 2019. https://www.fda.gov/news-events/speeches-fda-officials/breaking-down-barriers-between-clinical-trials-and-clinical-care-incorporating-real-world-evidence.

Haimovitch, Larry, and Richard Mark Kirkner. "A Look Behind Revision Optics' Shuttered Door." Ophthalmology Innovation Source (OIS), February 14, 2018. https://ois.net/look-behind-revision-optics-shuttered-door.

Hajat, Cother, and Emma Stein. "The Global Burden of Multiple Chronic Conditions: A Narrative Review." *Preventive Medicine Reports* 12 (2018): 284–93. https://doi.org/10.1016/j.pmedr.2018.10.008.

Harris, Sophie, Ari Miller, Stephanie Amiel, and Henrietta Mulnier. "Characterization of Adults with Type 1 Diabetes Not Attending Self-Management Education Courses: The Barriers to Uptake of Type 1 Diabetes Education (BUD1E) Study." *Qualitative Health Research* 29, no. 8 (2019): 1174–85. https://doi.org/10.1177/1049732318823718.

Harris, S. M., P. Shah, H. Mulnier, A. Healey, S. M. Thomas, S. A. Amiel, and D. Hopkins. "Factors Influencing Attendance at Structured Education for Type 1 Diabetes in South London." *Diabetic Medicine* 34, no. 6 (2017): 828–33. https://doi.org/10.1111/dme.13333.

Hartvigsen, Jan, Mark J. Hancock, Alice Kongsted, Quinette Louw, Manuela L. Ferreira, Stéphane Genevay, Damian Hoy, et al. "What Low Back Pain Is and Why We Need to Pay Attention." *Lancet* 391, no. 10137 (2018): 2356–67. https://doi.org/10.1016/S0140-6736(18)30480-X.

Health Sciences Authority. *Regulatory Guidelines for Software Medical Devices: A Lifecycle Approach.* Singapore: Health Sciences Authority, December 2019. https://www.hsa.gov.sg/docs/default-source/announcements/regulatory -updates/regulatory-guidelines-for-software-medical-devices--a-lifecycle -approach.pdf.

Hehner, Steffen, Stefan Biesdorf, and Manuel Möller. "Digitizing Healthcare— Opportunities for Germany." McKinsey & Company, October 31, 2018. https://www.mckinsey.com/industries/healthcare-systems-and-services /our-insights/digitizing-healthcare-opportunities-for-germany.

Henze, Stephanie, Amy Hung, Tobias Silberzahn, and Dandi Zhu. "Moving Digital Health Forward: Lessons on Business Building." McKinsey & Company, January 13, 2021. https://www.mckinsey.com/industries/life -sciences/our-insights/moving-digital-health-forward-lessons-on -business-building.

Heuvel, Roger van den, Nicolas G. Stamminger, Peter Mozerov, and Girisha Fernando. *Pathway to Success in Outcome-Based Contracting.* Zurich: KPMG Switzerland, 2020. https://assets.kpmg/content/dam/kpmg/ch /pdf/pathway-to-success-in-outcome-based-contracting.pdf.

Hood, Korey K., Marisa Hilliard, Gretchen Piatt, and Carolyn E. Ievers-Landis. "Effective Strategies for Encouraging Behavior Change in People with Diabetes." *Diabetes Management (London)* 5, no. 6 (2015): 499–510. https://www.ncbi.nlm.nih.gov/pmc/articles/PMC6086609.

Hoult, Molly. "Key Factors to Obtaining Reimbursement for Digital Therapeutics in the US." Eversana, February 4, 2021. https://www .eversana.com/insights/key-factors-to-obtaining-reimbursement-for -digital-therapeutics-in-the-u-s.

Howarth, Ana, Jose Quesada, Jessica Silva, Stephanie Judycki, and Peter R. Mills. "The Impact of Digital Health Interventions on Health-Related Outcomes in the Workplace: A Systematic Review." *Digital Health* 4 (2018). https://doi.org/10.1177/2055207618770861.

Huber, Stephan, Janosch A. Priebe, Kaja-Maria Baumann, Anne Plidschun, Christine Schiessl, and Thomas R. Tölle. "Treatment of Low Back Pain with a Digital Multidisciplinary Pain Treatment App: Short-Term Results." *JMIR Rehabilitation and Assistive Technologies* 4, no. 2 (2017): e11. https://doi.org/10.2196/rehab.9032.

Hult, Kristopher J. *Measuring the Potential Health Impact of Personalized Medicine: Evidence from Multiple Sclerosis Treatments.* Chicago: University of Chicago Press, 2019.

Humphreys, Gary. "Checklists Save Lives." *Bulletin of the World Health Organization* 86, no. 7 (2008): 501–2. https://doi.org/10.2471/BLT.08 .010708.

Hutchinson, Karen, Regina Sloutsky, Ashley Collimore, Benjamin Adams, Brian Harris, Terry D. Ellis, and Louis N. Awad. "A Music-Based Digital Therapeutic: Proof-of-Concept Automation of a Progressive and Individualized Rhythm-Based Walking Training Program after Stroke." *Neurorehabilitation and Neural Repair* 34, no. 11 (2020): 986–96. https://doi .org/10.1177/1545968320961114.

Iacoviello, Brian M., Joshua R. Steinerman, David B. Klein, Theodore L. Silver, Adam G. Berger, Sean X. Luo, and Nicholas J. Schork. "Clickotine, a Personalized Smartphone App for Smoking Cessation: Initial Evaluation." *JMIR mHealth and uHealth* 5, no. 4 (2017): e56. https://doi.org/10 .2196/mhealth.7226.

Institute for Clinical and Economic Review. "Cost-Effectiveness, the QALY, and the evLYG." Accessed November 1, 2021. https://icer.org /our-approach/methods-process/cost-effectiveness-the-qaly-and-the -evlyg.

Institute of Mental Health. "Singapore Residents Show a High Recognition of Diabetes, with Older People Being More Knowledgeable about the Condition." Media release, April 20, 2021. https://www.imh.com.sg /Newsroom/News-Releases/Documents/20Apr2021_Singapore resi- dents show a high recognition of diabetes.pdf.

Jacob, Christine, Antonio Sanchez-Vazquez, and Chris Ivory. "Social, Organizational, and Technological Factors Impacting Clinicians' Adoption of Mobile Health Tools: Systematic Literature Review." *JMIR mHealth and uHealth* 8, no. 2 (2020). https://doi.org/10.2196/15935.

Japsen, Bruce. "Inhaled Insulin's Cost May Take Breath Away." *Chicago Tribune*, February 1, 2006. https://www.chicagotribune.com/news/ct-xpm-2006-02-02-0602020156-story.html.

Johnson, Andrea. "Homepage Optimization." Marketing Experiments, March 23, 2016. https://marketingexperiments.com/a-b-testing/how-humana-optimized-banners.

Joyce, Rhod. *NHS Digital Health Technology Standard*. United Kingdom: National Health Service (NHS), February 24, 2020. https://assets.nhs.uk/prod/documents/NHS_Digital_Health_Technology_Standard_draft.pdf.

Kaplan, Warren, Veronika J. Wirtz, Aukje Mantel-Teeuwisse, Pieter Stolk, Béatrice Duthey, and Richard Laing. *Priority Medicines for Europe and the World: 2013 Update*. Geneva: World Health Organization, 2013. https://www.researchgate.net/publication/249995018_Priority_Medicines_for_Europe_and_the_World_2013_Update_Report.

Kasztura, Miriam, Aude Richard, Nefti-Eboni Bempong, Dejan Loncar, and Antoine Flahault. "Cost-Effectiveness of Precision Medicine: A Scoping Review." *International Journal of Public Health* 64 (December 2019): 1261–71. https://doi.org/10.1007/s00038-019-01298-x.

Kee, Theodore, Chee Weiyan, Agata Blasiak, Peter Wang, Jordan K. Chong, Jonna Chen, B. T. Thomas Yeo, Dean Ho, and Christopher L. Asplund. "Harnessing CURATE.AI as a Digital Therapeutics Platform by Identifying N-of-1 Learning Trajectory Profiles." *Advanced Therapeutics* 2, no. 9 (2019): 1900023. https://doi.org/10.1002/adtp.201900023.

Kennedy-Martin, Tessa, Kristina S. Boye, and Xiaomei Peng. "Cost of Medication Adherence and Persistence in Type 2 Diabetes Mellitus: A Literature Review." *Patient Preference and Adherence* 11 (2017): 1103–17. https://doi.org/10.2147/PPA.S136639.

Kennedy-Martin, Tessa, Sarah Curtis, Douglas Faries, Susan Robinson, and Joseph Johnston. "A Literature Review on the Representativeness of Randomized Controlled Trial Samples and Implications for the External Validity of Trial Results." *Trials* 16, no. 1 (2015): 1–14. https://doi.org/10.1186/s13063-015-1023-4.

Keown, Alex. "Sienna Biopharmaceuticals Files for Bankruptcy, Delaying Phase III Psoriasis Trial." BioSpace, September 18, 2019. https://www.biospace.com/article/sienna-biopharmaceuticals-files-chapter-11-delaying-phase-iii-psoriasis-trial.

Kerr, Ronny. "When Omada Health Was Young: The Early Years." *Vator TV*, March 21, 2017. https://vator.tv/news/2017-03-21-when-omada-health-was-young-the-early-years.

Kesavadev, Jothydev, Ashok Kumar Das, Ranjit Unnikrishnanlst, Sha-
shank R. Joshi, Ambady Ramachandran, Jisha Shamsudeen, Gopika
Krishnan, Sunitha Jothydev, and Viswanathan Mohan. "Use of Insulin
Pumps in India: Suggested Guidelines Based on Experience and Cultural
Differences." *Diabetes Technology & Therapeutics* 12, no. 10 (2010):
823–31. https://doi.org/10.1089/dia.2010.0027.

Kim, W. Chan, and Renée Mauborgne. *Blue Ocean Strategy: How to Create
Uncontested Market Space and Make the Competition Irrelevant.* Boston:
Harvard Business Review Press, 2015.

King, Kathryn M., Philip J. King, Rahul Nayar, and Scott Wilkes. "Perceptions of Adolescent Patients of the 'Lived Experience' of Type 1 Diabetes." *Diabetes Spectrum* 30, no. 1 (2017): 23–35. https://doi.org/10.2337
/ds15-0041.

Klonoff, David C., and David Kerr, "Overcoming Barriers to Adoption of
Digital Health Tools for Diabetes." *Journal of Diabetes Science and
Technology* 12, no. 1 (2018): 3–6. https://doi.org/10.1177/193229
6817732459.

Koh, Dean. "KT Signs MoU with Sibel Health to Expand Its Digital Health
Capabilities." *Mobihealth News*, November 12, 2020. https://www
.mobihealthnews.com/news/asia/kt-signs-mou-sibel-health-expand-its
-digital-health-capabilities.

Krist, Alex H., Sebastian T. Tong, Rebecca A. Aycock, and Daniel R. Longo.
"Engaging Patients in Decision-Making and Behavior Change to
Promote Prevention." *Studies in Health Technology and Informatics* 240
(2017): 284–302.

KT Corporation. "S.Korea's KT Corp. to Expand Digital Health Business
with Sibel." November 10, 2020. https://corp.kt.com/eng/html/promote
/news/report_detail.html?rows=10&page=1&datNo=16036.

Kyle Blankenship. "Camera Maker Kodak Dives into Drug Manufacturing
with $765M Federal Loan." *Fierce Pharma*, July 29, 2020. https://www
.fiercepharma.com/manufacturing/camera-maker-kodak-dives-into
-drug-manufacturing-765m-federal-loan.

Landi, Heather. "Teladoc's Virtual Visits Reach 3M during Q4 as Revenue
Grows to $383M." *Fierce Pharma*, February 25, 2021. https://www
.fiercehealthcare.com/tech/teladoc-s-virtual-visits-reach-3m-during-q4
-as-revenue-grows-to-383m.

Landi, Heather. "Telehealth Leader Teladoc to Buy Livongo in $18.5B Deal."
Fierce Healthcare, August 5, 2020. https://www.fiercehealthcare.com
/tech/teladoc-livongo-plan-to-merge-18-5b-deal.

Lerner, Jennifer S., Ye Li, Piercarlo Valdesolo, and Karim S. Kassam. "Emotion and Decision Making." *Annual Review of Psychology* 66 (January 2015): 799–823. https://doi.org/10.1146/annurev-psych-010213 -115043.

Levins, Hoag. "Report from the First National 'Nudge Units in Health Care' Symposium." University of Pennsylvania, Leonard Davis Institute of Health Economics, October 3, 2018. https://ldi.upenn.edu/our-work /research-updates/report-from-the-first-national-nudge-units-in-health -care-symposium.

Liu, Xiaoxuan, Livia Faes, Aditya U. Kale, Siegfried K. Wagner, Dun Jack Fu, Alice Bruynseels, Thushika Mahendiran, et al. "A Comparison of Deep Learning Performance against Health-Care Professionals in Detecting Diseases from Medical Imaging: A Systematic Review and Meta-Analysis." *Lancet Digital Health* 1, no. 6 (2019): e271–97. https://doi .org/10.1016/S2589-7500(19)30123-2.

Livongo Health. "Livongo Reports Third Quarter 2020 Financial Results." *Globe Newswire*, October 28, 2020. https://www.globenewswire.com /news-release/2020/10/28/2116285/0/en/Livongo-Reports-Third -Quarter-2020-Financial-Results.html.

Livongo Health. "United States Securities and Exchange Commission Form S-1 Registration Statement." Filed on June 28, 2019. Registration No. 333-. https://www.sec.gov/Archives/edgar/data/1639225/00011 9312519185159/d731249ds1.htm.

Lorenzoni, Luca, Alberto Marino, David Morgan, and Chris James. *Health Spending Projections to 2030: New Results Based on a Revised OECD Methodology.* OECD Health Working Papers No. 110. Paris: OECD Publishing, 2019. https://doi.org/10.1787/5667f23d-en.

Luo, Candice, Nitika Sanger, Nikhita Singhal, Kaitlin Pattrick, Ieta Shams, Hamnah Shahid, Peter Hoang, et al. "A Comparison of Electronically Delivered and Face-to-Face Cognitive Behavioural Therapies in Depressive Disorders: A Systematic Review and Meta-Analysis." *eClinical Medicine* 24 (2020). https://doi.org/10.1016/j.eclinm.2020.100442.

Manta, Christine, Bray Patrick-Lake, and Jennifer C. Goldsack. "Digital Measures that Matter to Patients: A Framework to Guide the Selection and Development of Digital Measures of Health." *Digital Biomarkers* 4, no. 3 (2020): 69–77. https://doi.org/10.1159/000509725.

Marshall, Sheila K. "Do I Matter? Construct Validation of Adolescents' Perceived Mattering to Parents and Friends." *Journal of Adolescence* 24, no. 4 (2001): 473–90. https://doi.org/10.1006/jado.2001.0384.

Marshall, Sheila K., and Lauree Tilton-Weaver. "Adolescents' Perceived Mattering to Parents and Friends: Testing Cross-Lagged Associations with Psychosocial Well-Being." *International Journal of Behavioral Development* 43, no. 6 (2019): 541–52. https://doi.org/10.1177 /0165025419844019.

Martino, Maureen, Liz Jones Hollis, and Erica Teichert. "Pharma's Biggest Flops." *Fierce Pharma*, October 18, 2020. https://www.fiercepharma.com /special-report/exubera-pharma-s-biggest-flops.

Matera, Camilla, Nicolina Bosco, and Patrizia Meringolo. "Perceived Mattering to Family and Friends, Self-Esteem, and Well-Being." *Psychology, Health & Medicine* 25, no. 5 (2020): 550–58. https://doi.org/10.1080 /13548506.2019.1626454.

Mathews, Anna W., and Danny Yadron. "Health Insurer Anthem Hit by Hackers." *Wall Street Journal*, February 4, 2015. https://www.wsj.com /articles/health-insurer-anthem-hit-by-hackers-1423103720.

McCarthy, Owen. "Looking Back & Ahead at the Digital Therapeutics Industry." *Medium*, December 23, 2020. https://medrhythms.medium .com/looking-back-ahead-at-the-digital-therapeutics-industry -2e8454d342c5.

McGlynn, Elizabeth A., Steven M. Asch, John Adams, Joan Keesey, Jennifer Hicks, Alison DeCristofaro, and Eve A. Kerr. "The Quality of Health Care Delivered to Adults in the United States." *New England Journal of Medicine* 348, no. 26 (2003): 2635–45. https://doi.org/10.1056 /NEJMsa022615.

McGrath, Rita Gunter, and Ian C. MacMillan. "Discovery-Driven Planning." *Harvard Business Review*, July–August 1995. https://hbr.org/1995 /07/discovery-driven-planning.

McIntyre, Harold David, "Dose Adjustment for Normal Eating: A Role for the Expert Patient?" *Diabetes & Metabolism Journal* 38, no. 2 (2014): 87–91. https://doi.org/10.4093/dmj.2014.38.2.87.

MedRhythms. "MedRhythms Announces an Expansion of Intellectual Property Portfolio, Securing Patent on Audio Engine for Digital Therapeutics Platform." *Cision PR Newswire*, April 17, 2020. https://www .prnewswire.com/news-releases/medrhythms-announces-an-expansion -of-intellectual-property-portfolio-securing-patent-on-audio-engine -for-digital-therapeutics-platform-301042485.html.

"Medtronic Profit Margin 2006–2021." *Macrotrends*, accessed July 31, 2021. https://www.macrotrends.net/stocks/charts/MDT/medtronic/profit -margins.

Megginson, Leon C. "Lessons from Europe for American Business." *South-western Social Science Quarterly* 44, no. 1 (1963): 3–13. http://www.jstor.org/stable/42866937.

Mehra, Mandeep R., Sapan S. Desai, Frank Ruschitzka, and Amit N. Patel. "Retracted: Hydroxychloroquine or Chloroquine with or without a Macrolide for Treatment of COVID-19: A Multinational Registry Analysis." *Lancet*, May 22, 2020. https://doi.org/10.1016/S0140-6736(20)31180-6.

Michie, Susan, Robert West, Kate Sheals, and Cristina A. Godinho. "Evaluating the Effectiveness of Behavior Change Techniques in Health-Related Behavior: A Scoping Review of Methods Used." *Translational Behavioral Medicine* 8, no. 2 (2018): 212–24. https://doi.org/10.1093/tbm/ibx019.

Miliard, Mike. "AMA Sees Surge in Health IT Adoption, 'Rise of the Digital-Native Physician.'" *Healthcare IT News*, February 6, 2020. https://www.healthcareitnews.com/news/ama-sees-surge-health-it-adoption-rise-digital-native-physician.

Mobiquity Inc. "COVID-19: Ensuring a Quality Patient Experience with the Rise of Digitisation in a Healthcare Setting." Mobiquity, January 21, 2021. https://www.mobiquity.com/insights/covid-19-research-study-digital-health-report-2021.

Moller, Arlen C., Gina Merchant, David E. Conroy, Robert West, Eric Hekler, Kari C. Kugler, and Susan Michie. "Applying and Advancing Behavior Change Theories and Techniques in the Context of a Digital Health Revolution: Proposals for More Effectively Realizing Untapped Potential." *Journal of Behavioral Medicine* 40 (February 2017): 85–98. https://doi.org/10.1007/s10865-016-9818-7.

Muoio, Dave. "BlueStar's Eighth FDA Clearance Adds Long-Acting Basal Insulin Support for Type 2 Patients." *Mobihealth News*, June 3, 2020. https://www.mobihealthnews.com/news/bluestars-eighth-fda-clearance-adds-long-acting-basal-insulin-support-type-2-patients.

Muoio, Dave. "Proteus Parts Ways with Otsuka as It Pivots toward Oncology, Infectious Disease Treatment Adherence." *Mobihealth News*, January 14, 2020. https://www.mobihealthnews.com/news/proteus-parts-ways-otsuka-it-pivots-toward-oncology-infectious-disease-treatment-adherence.

Murray, Elizabeth, Eric B. Hekler, Gerhard Andersson, Linda M. Collins, Aiden Doherty, Chris Hollis, Daniel E. Rivera, Robert West, and Jeremy C. Wyatt. "Evaluating Digital Health Interventions: Key Questions and Approaches." *American Journal of Preventive Medicine* 51, no. 5 (2016): 843–51. https://doi.org/10.1016/j.amepre.2016.06.008.

Naser, Abdallah Y., Anas Nawfal Hameed, Nour Mustafa, Hassan Alwafi, Eman Zmaily Dahmash, Hamad S. Alyami, and Haya Khalil. "Depression and Anxiety in Patients With Cancer: A Cross-Sectional Study." *Frontiers in Psychology* 12 (2021): 585534. https://doi.org/10.3389/fpsyg.2021.585534.

National Cancer Institute at the National Institutes of Health. "Standard of Care." 2021. https://www.cancer.gov/publications/dictionaries/cancer-terms/def/standard-of-care.

National Center for Advancing Translational Sciences. "About NCATS." Accessed September 23, 2021. https://ncats.nih.gov/about.

National Human Genome Research Institute. "Rare Diseases FAQ." Accessed January 26, 2021. https://www.genome.gov/FAQ/Rare-Diseases.

National Institute for Health and Care Excellence (NICE). *Continuous Subcutaneous Insulin Infusion for the Treatment of Diabetes Mellitus: Technology Appraisal Guidance.* London: NICE, 2008. https://www.nice.org.uk/guidance/TA151.

National Institute for Health and Care Excellence (NICE). *Evidence Standards Framework for Digital Health Technologies.* London: NICE, March 2019. https://www.nice.org.uk/Media/Default/About/what-we-do/our-programmes/evidence-standards-framework/digital-evidence-standards-framework.pdf.

National Medical Research Council. *Diabetes Taskforce Report.* Singapore: Ministry of Health, 2020. https://www.nmrc.gov.sg/docs/default-source/about-us-library/dtf-summary-report.pdf.

Naujokaite, Ruta. "What is the Digital Care Act (DVG)?" *Chino.io Blog*, June 23, 2020. https://www.chino.io/blog/what-is-the-digital-care-act-dvg.

Noell, Guillaume, Rosa Faner, and Alvar Agustí. "From Systems Biology to P4 Medicine: Applications in Respiratory Medicine." *European Respiratory Review* 27, no. 147 (2018). https://doi.org/10.1183/16000617.0110-2017.

OCEBM Levels of Evidence Working Group. "The Oxford 2011 Levels of Evidence." Centre for Evidence-Based Medicine (CEBM). Accessed November 17, 2022. https://www.cebm.ox.ac.uk/resources/levels-of-evidence/ocebm-levels-of-evidence.

Omada Health. "Omada Digital Diabetes Prevention Program Shows Sustained HbA1c Reduction and Weight Loss in Randomized Control Trial." *Cision PR Newswire*, November 3, 2020. https://www.prnewswire.com/news-releases/omada-digital-diabetes-prevention-program-shows

-sustained-hba1c-reduction-and-weight-loss-in-randomized-control
-trial-301165318.html.

Organisation for Economic Co-operation and Development (OECD).
"Employment Rate." OECD Data, accessed November 17, 2022. https://
data.oecd.org/emp/employment-rate.htm.

Organisation for Economic Co-operation and Development (OECD). *Health
at a Glance 2011: OECD Indicators.* Paris: OECD Publishing, 2011. https://
www.oecd.org/els/health-systems/49105858.pdf.

Organisation for Economic Co-operation and Development (OECD).
Out-of-Pocket Spending: Access to Care and Financial Protection. Paris:
OECD, April 2019. https://www.oecd.org/health/health-systems/OECD
-Focus-on-Out-of-Pocket-Spending-April-2019.pdf.

Pantuck, Allan J., Dong-Keun Lee, Theodore Kee, Peter Wang, Sanjay
Lakhotia, Michael H. Silverman, Colleen Mathis, et al. "Modulating BET
Bromodomain Inhibitor ZEN-3694 and Enzalutamide Combination
Dosing in a Metastatic Prostate Cancer Patient Using CURATE.AI, an
Artificial Intelligence Platform." *Advanced Therapeutics* 1, no. 6 (2018).
https://doi.org/10.1002/adtp.201800104.

Parcher, Benjamin, and Megan Coder. "Decision Makers Need an Approach
to Determine Digital Therapeutic Product Quality, Access, and Appropriate Use." *Journal of Managed Care & Specialty Pharmacy* 27, no. 4
(2021): 536–38. https://doi.org/10.18553/jmcp.2021.27.4.536.

Pear Therapeutics. "Clinical Evidence." reSET-O and reSET Proven Outcomes, 2021. https://resetforrecovery.com/outcomes/.

Pear Therapeutics. "Pear Therapeutics Closes $20 Million Financing." Press
release, accessed November 17, 2022. https://peartherapeutics.com/pear
-therapeutics-raises-20-million-to-launch-a-family-of-prescription
-digital-therapies-treating-disorders-of-the-brain.

Pear Therapeutics. "Reset for Recovery: The Proof." Accessed November, 11,
2022. https://www.resetforrecovery.com/reset#the-proof.

Peyrot, Mark, R. R. Rubin, T. Lauritzen, F. J. Snoek, D. R. Matthews, and
S. E. Skovlund. "Psychosocial Problems and Barriers to Improved
Diabetes Management: Results of the Cross-National Diabetes Attitudes, Wishes and Needs (DAWN) Study." *Diabetic Medicine* 22, no. 10
(2005): 1379–85. https://doi.org/10.1111/j.1464-5491.2005.01644.x.

Pichai, Sundar. "Privacy Should Not Be a Luxury Good." *New York
Times*, May 7, 2019. https://www.nytimes.com/2019/05/07/opinion
/google-sundar-pichai-privacy.html.

Piller, Charles, and Kelly Servick. "Two Elite Medical Journals Retract Coronavirus Papers over Data Integrity Questions." *Science*, June 4, 2020. https://www.science.org/news/2020/06/two-elite-medical -journals-retract-coronavirus-papers-over-data-integrity-questions.

Ping An. *2020 Annual Report*. Shenzhen: Ping An, February 3, 2021. https://group.pingan.com/resource/pingan/IR-Docs/2020/pingan-ar20 -report.pdf.

Ping An. *Announcement of Unaudited Results for the Three Months Ended March 31, 2020*. Shenzhen: Ping An, April 23, 2020. https://doc.irasia .com/listco/hk/pingan/announcement/a228455-e_02318ann _20200423(20200423_1445).pdf.

Ping An. "Ping An Good Doctor Has Become the First Online Healthcare Platform with More Than 300 Million Registered Users." *Cision PR Newswire*, September 23, 2019. https://www.prnewswire.com/news -releases/ping-an-good-doctor-has-become-the-first-online-healthcare -platform-with-more-than-300-million-registered-users-300923026.html.

Ping An. "Ping An Unveils Health Care Ecosystem Strategy." *Cision PR Newswire*, September 23, 2020. https://www.prnewswire.com/news-releases /ping-an-unveils-health-care-ecosystem-strategy-301136665.html.

Piper, Megan E., Michael C. Fiore, Stevens S. Smith, David Fraser, Daniel M. Bolt, Linda M. Collins, Robin Mermelstein, et al. "Identifying Effective Intervention Components for Smoking Cessation: A Factorial Screening Experiment." *Addiction* 111, no. 1 (2016): 129–41. https://doi .org/10.1111/add.13162.

Plsek, Paul. "Redesigning Health Care with Insights from the Science of Complex Adaptive Systems." In *Crossing the Quality Chasm: A New Health Care System for the 21st Century*, edited by Institute of Medicine Committee on Quality of Health Care in America, 309–22. Washington, DC: National Academy Press, 2001.

Prabhu, Nishitha, and Parvathy R. Menon. "Express Scripts a Pioneer: Launches Curated List of Digital Therapeutics." Clarivate, December 12, 2019. https://clarivate.com/blog/express-scripts-pioneer-launches -curated-list-digital-therapeutics.

Precedence Research. "Digital Therapeutics Market Size to Hit US$ 11.82 Bn by 2027." *Globe Newswire*, October 19, 2020. https://www.globe newswire.com/news-release/2020/10/19/2110561/0/en/Digital -Therapeutics-Market-Size-to-Hit-US-11-82-Bn-by-2027.html.

Priebe, Janosch A., Katharina K. Haas, Leida F. Moreno Sanchez, Karin Schoefmann, Daniel A. Utpadel-Fischler, Paul Stockert, Reinhard

Thoma, et al. "Digital Treatment of Back Pain versus Standard of Care: The Cluster-Randomized Controlled Trial, Rise-uP." *Journal of Pain Research* 13 (2020): 1823–38. https://doi.org/10.2147/JPR.S260761.

Ravot, Elisabetta, and Roberto Ascione. "Access/Reimbursement Policies for Digital Therapeutics Already in Use in National Health Systems." *Tendenze nuove*, Special Issue 4 (2021): 105–16. https://www.tenden zenuove.it/2021/07/29/access-reimbursement-policies-for-digital -therapeutics-already-in-use-in-national-health-systems.

Resnikoff, Serge, Van Charles Lansingh, Lindsey Washburn, William Felch, Tina-Marie Gauthier, Hugh R. Taylor, Kristen Eckert, David Parke, and Peter Wiedemann. "Estimated Number of Ophthalmologists Worldwide (International Council of Ophthalmology Update): Will We Meet the Needs?" *British Journal of Ophthalmology* 104, no. 4 (2020): 588–92. https://doi.org/10.1136/bjophthalmol-2019-314336.

Reuter, Elise. "Proteus Files for Bankruptcy: Where Did It Falter?" *MedCity News*, June 16, 2020. https://medcitynews.com/2020/06/proteus-files -for-bankruptcy-where-did-it-falter.

Riddle, Matthew C., Julio Rosenstock, and John Gerich, "The Treat-to-Target Trial: Randomized Addition of Glargine or Human NPH Insulin to Oral Therapy of Type 2 Diabetic Patients." *Diabetes Care* 26, no. 11 (2003): 3080–86. https://doi.org/10.2337/diacare.26.11.3080.

Robbins, Michele, Janice Tufte, and Clarissa Hsu. "Learning to 'Swim' with the Experts: Experiences of Two Patient Co-Investigators for a Project Funded by the Patient-Centered Outcomes Research Institute." *Permanente Journal* 20, no. 2 (2016): 85–88. https://doi.org/10 .7812/TPP/15-162.

Roehl, Michael Joseph. "DiGA: Digital Therapeutics in Germany." *LinkedIn*, March 9, 2022. https://www.linkedin.com/pulse/diga-digital-therapeutics -germany-michael-joseph-roehl.

Ross, Jamie, Fiona Stevenson, Rosa Lau, and Elizabeth Murray. "Factors that Influence the Implementation of e-Health: A Systematic Review of Systematic Reviews (An Update)." *Implementation Science* 11, no. 1 (2016): 1–12. https://doi.org/10.1186/s13012-016-0510-7.

Rossignol, S., and G. Melvill Jones. "Audio-Spinal Influence in Man Studied by the H-Reflex and Its Possible Role on Rhythmic Movements Synchronized to Sound." *Electroencephalography and Clinical Neurophysiology* 41, no. 1 (1976): 83–92. https://doi.org/10.1016/0013-4694(76)90217-0.

Rubin, Devon I. "Epidemiology and Risk Factors for Spine Pain." *Neurologic Clinics* 25, no. 2 (2007): 353–71. https://doi.org/10.1016/j.ncl.2007.01.004.

Sanofi. "Sanofi and Abbott Partner to Integrate Glucose Sensing and Insulin Delivery Technologies to Help Change the Way Diabetes Is Managed." Press release, September 16, 2019. https://www.sanofi.com/en/media-room/press-releases/2019/2019-09-16-07-00-00.

Savonix, "Savonix and Boston University School of Public Health Launch Landmark Population Health Alzheimer's Disease Discovery Study (ASSIST) to Digitally Collect Brain Health Data." *Businesswire*, November 04, 2019. https://www.businesswire.com/news/home/20191104005287/en/Savonix-and-Boston-University-School-of-Public-Health-Launch-Landmark-Population-Health-Alzheimer's-Disease-Discovery-Study-ASSIST-to-Digitally-Collect-Brain-Health-Data.

Savnoix. "Savonix and Fujitsu Connected Technologies Limited Partner to Introduce Savonix Mobile App on Raku-Raku Smartphone F-42A." *Businesswire*, September 29, 2020. https://www.businesswire.com/news/home/20200929005016/en/Savonix-and-Fujitsu-Connected-Technologies-Limited-Partner-to-Introduce-Savonix-Mobile-App-on-Raku-Raku-Smartphone-F-42A.

"Scailyte among the Spinoff Finalists for the Global Nature Research Awards." Swiss Biotech, June 20, 2020. https://www.swissbiotech.org/listing/scailyte-among-the-spinoff-prize-finalists.

Shah, Nigam H., Arnold Milstein, and Steven C. Bagley. "Making Machine Learning Models Clinically Useful." *JAMA* 322, no. 14 (2019): 1351–52. https://doi.org/10.1001/jama.2019.10306.

Sham, Julian. *Accenture 2019 Digital Health Consumer Survey: Singapore Results*. Accenture Health, 2019. https://www.accenture.com/_acnmedia/pdf-102/accenture-digital-health-consumer-survey-singapore.pdf.

Shen, Yinzhong, Tingyi Liu, Jun Chen, Xin Li, Li Liu, Jiayin Shen, Jiangrong Wang, et al. "Harnessing Artificial Intelligence to Optimize Long-Term Maintenance Dosing for Antiretroviral-Naive Adults with HIV-1 Infection." *Advanced Therapeutics* 3, no. 4 (2019): 1900114. https://doi.org/10.1002/adtp.201900114.

Sherwin, Robert S., Robert M. Anderson, John B. Buse, Marshall H. Chin, David Eddy, Judith Fradkin, Theodore G. Ganiats, et al. "The Prevention or Delay of Type 2 Diabetes." Supplement, *Diabetes Care* 26, no. S1 (2003): S62–69. https://doi.org/10.2337/diacare.26.2007.S62.

Singapore Ministry of Health. "National Health Survey 2010." November 2011. https://www.moh.gov.sg/resources-statistics/reports/national-health-survey-2010.

Singapore News Center. "Zuellig Pharma Shapes the Future of Healthcare with the Cloud." Microsoft, August 26, 2019. https://news.microsoft .com/en-sg/2019/08/26/zuellig-pharma-shapes-the-future-of -healthcare-with-the-cloud/.

Singapore Statutes Online. "Health Products Act 2007." Accessed March 1, 2021. https://sso.agc.gov.sg/Act/HPA2007.

Sinsky, Christine, Lacey Colligan, Ling Li, Mirela Prgomet, Sam Reynolds, Lindsey Goeders, Johanna Westbrook, Michael Tutty, and George Blike. "Allocation of Physician Time in Ambulatory Practice: A Time and Motion Study in 4 Specialties." *Annals of Internal Medicine* 165, no. 11 (2016): 753–60. https://doi.org/10.7326/M16-0961.

Speich, Benjamin, Belinda von Niederhäusern, Nadine Schur, Lars G. Hemkens, Thomas Fürst, Neera Bhatnagar, Reem Alturki, et al. "Systematic Review on Costs and Resource Use of Randomized Clinical Trials Shows a Lack of Transparent and Comprehensive Data." *Journal of Clinical Epidemiology* 96 (2018): 1–11. https://doi.org/10.1016/j.jclinepi.2017.12.018.

States, Rebecca A., Evangelos Pappas, and Yasser Salem. "Overground Physical Therapy Gait Training for Chronic Stroke Patients with Mobility Deficits." *Cochrane Database of Systematic Reviews*, no. 3 (2009): CD006075. https://doi.org/10.1002/14651858.CD006075.pub2.

Staton, Tracy. "The Top 10 Patent Losses of 2015." *Fierce Pharma*, December 17, 2014. https://www.fiercepharma.com/special-report/abilify-0.

Stern, Theodore A., Gregory L. Fricchione, and Jerrold F. Rosenbaum, *Massachusetts General Hospital Handbook of General Hospital Psychiatry*. Elsevier Health Sciences, 2010. https://doi.org/10.1016/B978-1-4377 -1927-7.00003-0.

STL Partners. "Four Strategies for Telcos in Healthcare." Accessed November 17, 2022. https://stlpartners.com/digital-health-telecoms/four -strategies-for-telcos-in-healthcare.

Subramaniam, M., E. Abdin, L. Picco, S. Pang, S. Shafie, J.A. Vaingankar, K. W. Kwok, K. Verma, and S. A. Chong. "Stigma towards People with Mental Disorders and Its Components: A Perspective from Multi-Ethnic Singapore." *Epidemiology and Psychiatric Sciences* 26, no. 4 (2017): 371–82.

Szajewska, Hania. "Evidence-Based Medicine and Clinical Research: Both Are Needed, Neither Is Perfect." *Annals of Nutrition and Metabolism* 72, no. suppl_3 (2018): 13–23. https://doi.org/10.1159/000487375.

Teladoc Health. "Teladoc Health and Livongo Merge to Create New Standard in Global Healthcare Delivery, Access and Experience." Press release,

August 5, 2020. https://www.teladochealth.com/newsroom/press
/release/Teladoc-Health-and-Livongo-Merge-to-Create-New-Standard
-in-Global-Healthcare-Delivery-Access-and-Experience-08-05-2020.

Teladoc Health. "Teladoc Health Reports Third-Quarter 2020 Results."
Press release, October 28, 2020. https://ir.teladochealth.com/news-and
-events/investor-news/press-release-details/2020/Teladoc-Health
-Reports-Third-Quarter-2020-Results/default.aspx.

Teladoc Health. "Teladoc Health to Announce Third Quarter 2022 Financial Results." Press release, October 11, 2022. https://ir.teladochealth
.com/news-and-events/investor-news/press-release-details/2022
/Teladoc-Health-to-Announce-Third-Quarter-2022-Financial-Results
/default.aspx.

Thielbar, Kelly O., Kristen M. Triandafilou, Alexander J. Barry, Ning Yuan,
Arthur Nishimoto, Joelle Johnson, Mary Ellen Stoykov, Daria Tsoup-
ikova, and Derek G. Kamper. "Home-Based Upper Extremity Stroke
Therapy Using a Multiuser Virtual Reality Environment: A Randomized
Trial." *Archives of Physical Medicine and Rehabilitation* 101, no. 2, 196–203.
https://doi.org/10.1016/j.apmr.2019.10.182.

TM Forum. "Telco Cloud Orchestration Plus, Using Open API on IoT."
Accessed November 17, 2022. https://www.tmforum.org/collaboration
/catalyst-program/telco-cloud-orchestration-plus-using-open-api-iot.

Toelle, Thomas R., Daniel A. Utpadel-Fischler, Katharina-Kristina Haas,
and Janosch A. Priebe. "App-Based Multidisciplinary Back Pain Treatment versus Combined Physiotherapy Plus Online Education: A Randomized Controlled Trial." *NPJ Digital Medicine* 2 (May 2019): 1–9.
https://doi.org/10.1038/s41746-019-0109-x.

Toh, Ee Ming, and Wong Pei Ting. "The Big Read: Apathy, Complacency—
the Worst Enemies in Singapore's War against Diabetes." *Today*, August 25, 2017. https://www.todayonline.com/singapore/apathy
-complacency-worst-enemies-in-war-against-diabetes.

Trimble, Michael, and Dale Hesdorffer. "Music and the Brain: The Neuroscience of Music and Musical Appreciation." *BJPsych International* 14,
no. 2 (2017): 28–31. https://doi.org/10.1192/s2056474000001720.

Trzeciak, Stephen, and Anthony Mazzarelli. *Compassionomics: The Revolutionary Scientific Evidence that Caring Makes a Difference.* Pensacola, FL:
Studer Group, 2019.

UCB Biopharma. "Study to Evaluate the Impact of Using Wearable Devices
in Addition to Standard Clinical Practice on Parkinson's Subject Symp-

toms Management." ClinicalTrials.gov, February 19, 2019. https://
clinicaltrials.gov/ct2/show/NCT03103919.

UpScripts Somryst. "Train Your Brain for Better Sleep." Accessed November 17, 2022. https://www.sleepdocconsult.com/products/somryst-for
-chronic-insomnia.

US Food and Drug Administration. "Artificial Intelligence and Machine
Learning in Software as a Medical Device." Accessed January 12, 2021.
https://www.fda.gov/medical-devices/software-medical-device-samd
/artificial-intelligence-and-machine-learning-software-medical
-device#regulation.

US Food and Drug Administration. "De Novo Classification Request."
Accessed November 20, 2019. https://www.fda.gov/medical-devices
/premarket-submissions/de-novo-classification-request.

US Food and Drug Administration. "Digital Health Software Precertification (Pre-Cert) Pilot Program." Accessed May 6, 2019. https://www.fda
.gov/medical-devices/digital-health-center-excellence/digital-health
-software-precertification-pre-cert-program.

US Food and Drug Administration. "Investigational Device Exemption
(IDE)." Accessed December 13, 2019. https://www.fda.gov/medical
-devices/how-study-and-market-your-device/investigational-device
-exemption-ide.

US Food and Drug Administration. "Premarket Approval (PMA)." May 16,
2019. https://www.fda.gov/medical-devices/premarket-submissions
/premarket-approval-pma.

US Food and Drug Administration. "Premarket Notification 510(k)."
Accessed March 13, 2020. https://www.fda.gov/medical-devices
/premarket-submissions/premarket-notification-510k.

US Food and Drug Administration. *Use of Real-World Evidence to Support
Regulatory Decision-Making for Medical Devices: Guidance for Industry and
Food and Drug Administration Staff.* Silver Spring, MD: FDA, August 31,
2017. https://www.fda.gov/media/99447/download.

Van Oostrom, Sandra H., H. Susan J. Picavet, Simone R. de Bruin, Irina
Stirbu, Joke C. Korevaar, Francois G. Schellevis, and Caroline A. Baan.
"Multimorbidity of Chronic Diseases and Health Care Utilization in
General Practice." *BMC Family Practice* 15, no. 1 (2014): 1–9. https://doi
.org/10.1186/1471-2296-15-61.

Verghese, Joe, Roee Holtzer, Richard B. Lipton, and Cuiling Wang. "Quantitative Gait Markers and Incident Fall Risk in Older Adults." *Journals of*

Gerontology: Series A 64A, no. 8 (2009): 896–901. https://doi.org/10.1093 /gerona/glp033.

Vohra, Sunita, Larissa Shamseer, Margaret Sampson, Cecilia Bukutu, Christopher H. Schmid, Robyn Tate, Jane Nikles, Deborah R. Zucker, Richard Kravitz, Gordon Guyatt, Douglas G. Altman, and David Moher. "CONSORT Extension for Reporting N-of-1 Trials (CENT) 2015 Statement." *BMJ* 350 (2015). https://doi.org/10.1136/bmj.h1738.

Volk, JoAnn, Dania Palanker, Madeline O'Brien, Christina L. Goe. "States' Actions to Expand Telemedicine Access during COVID-19 and Future Policy Considerations." The Commonwealth Fund, June 23, 2021. https://www.commonwealthfund.org/publications/issue-briefs/2021 /jun/states-actions-expand-telemedicine-access-covid-19.

Voyer, Benjamin G. "'Nudging' Behaviours in Healthcare: Insights from Behavioural Economics." *British Journal of Healthcare Management* 21, no. 3 (2015): 130–35. https://doi.org/10.12968/bjhc.2015.21.3.130.

"VP Live." Virgin Pulse. Accessed November 17, 2022. https://community .virginpulse.com/vp-live-shortlister.

Wei, Khor Ing. "Nurture or Nature? Research Project Reveals Answers." *MediCine*, no. 27 (2018): 18–19. https://medicine.nus.edu.sg/wp-content /uploads/2018/08/MediCine_Issue27.pdf.

Welldoc Inc. "Welldoc Receives FDA Clearance for Long-Acting Insulin Support for Award-Winning Digital Health Solution BlueStar." *Cision PR Newswire*, June 3, 2020. https://www.prnewswire.com/news-releases /welldoc-receives-fda-clearance-for-long-acting-insulin-support-for -award-winning-digital-health-solution-bluestar-301069807.html.

Welldoc Inc. "WellDoc Validates Potential of Its Digital Therapeutic, BlueStar, to Significantly Reduce Healthcare Costs," *Global Newswire*, January 4, 2008. https://www.globenewswire.com/en/news-release /2018/01/04/1283402/36511/en/WellDoc-Validates-Potential-of-Its -Digital-Therapeutic-BlueStar-to-Significantly-Reduce-Healthcare-Costs .html.

Wenger, Nathalie, Marie Méan, Julien Castioni, Pedro Marques-Vidal, Gérard Waeber, and Antoine Garnier. "Allocation of Internal Medicine Resident Time in a Swiss Hospital: A Time and Motion Study of Day and Evening Shifts." *Annals of Internal Medicine* 166, no. 8 (2017): 579–86. https://doi.org/10.7326/M16-2238.

Whaley, Christopher M., Jennifer B. Bollyky, Wei Lu, Stefanie Painter, Jennifer Schneider, Zhenxiang Zhao, Xuanyao He, Jennal Johnson, and Eric S. Meadows. "Reduced Medical Spending Associated with

Increased Use of a Remote Diabetes Management Program and Lower Mean Blood Glucose Values." *Journal of Medical Economics* 22, no. 9 (2019): 869–77. https://doi.org/10.1080/13696998.2019.1609483.

Wientraub, Arlene. "Pfizer's Exubera Flop." *Bloomberg*, October 18, 2007. https://www.bloomberg.com/news/articles/2007-10-18/pfizers-exubera-flopbusinessweek-business-news-stock-market-and-financial-advice.

World Health Organization. *Adherence to Long-Term Therapies: Evidence for Action*. Geneva: WHO, 2003. https://apps.who.int/iris/handle/10665/42682.

World Health Organization. "Asthma: Key Facts." Accessed March 3, 2021. https://www.who.int/news-room/fact-sheets/detail/asthma.

World Health Organization. "Cardiovascular Diseases (CVDs)." June 11, 2021. http://www.who. int/mediacentre/factsheets/fs317/en/index.html.

World Health Organization. "Dementia: Key Facts." September 20, 2022. https://www.who.int/news-room/fact-sheets/detail/dementia.

World Health Organization, "Diabetes: Key Facts." Accessed April 13, 2021. https://www.who.int/news-room/fact-sheets/detail/diabetes.

World Health Organization. *Global Strategic Directions for Strengthening Nursing and Midwifery 2016–2020*. Geneva: World Health Organization, 2016. https://apps.who.int/iris/rest/bitstreams/1157318/retrieve.

World Health Organization. "The Top 10 Causes of Death." December 9, 2020. https://www.who.int/news-room/fact-sheets/detail/the-top-10-causes-of-death.

World Health Organization. "WHO Director-General's Opening Remarks at the Media Briefing on COVID-19." May 25, 2020. https://www.who.int/director-general/speeches/detail/who-director-general-s-opening-remarks-at-the-media-briefing-on-covid-19---25-may-2020.

Wu, Aimin, Lyn March, Xuanqi Zheng, Jinfeng Huang, Xiangyang Wang, Jie Zhao, Fiona M. Blyth, Emma Smith, Rachelle Buchbinder, and Damian Hoy. "Global Low Back Pain Prevalence and Years Lived with Disability from 1990 to 2017: Estimates from the Global Burden of Disease Study 2017." *Annals of Translational Medicine* 8, no. 6 (2020): 299. https://doi.org/10.21037/atm.2020.02.175.

Yonhap. "Telcos Expand Digital Health Care Services amid Pandemic." *Korea Herald*, September 14, 2020. http://www.koreaherald.com/view.php?ud=20200914000919.

Young, Scott W. H. "Improving Library User Experience with A/B Testing: Principles and Process." *Weave: Journal of Library User Experience* 1, no. 1 (2014). https://doi.org/10.3998/weave.12535642.0001.101.

Zaleha H, S., Nora Ithnin, Nur Haliza Abdul Wahab, and Noorhazirah Sunar. "Intelligent Locking System Using Deep Learning for Autonomous Vehicle in Internet of Things." *International Journal of Advanced Computer Science and Applications* 12, no. 10 (2021): 565–78. http://dx.doi.org/10.14569/IJACSA.2021.0121063.

Zarrinpar, A., Lee, D. K., Silva, A., Datta, N., Kee, T., Eriksen, C., Weigle, K., Agopian, V., Kaldas, F., Farmer, D., Wang, S. E., Busuttil, R., Ho, C. M., & Ho, D. "Individualizing Liver Transplant Immunosuppression Using a Phenotypic Personalized Medicine Platform." *Science Translational Medicine* 8, no. 333 (2016). https://doi.org/10.1126/scitranslmed.aac5954.

Zelinka, Ivan, Thanh Cong Truong, Diep Quoc Bao, Lumir Kojecky, and Eslam Amer. "Artificial Intelligence in Astrophysics." In *Intelligent Astrophysics*, edited by Ivan Zelinka, Massimo Brescia, and Dalya Baron, 1–28. Cham, Switzerland: Springer Nature, 2021.

Big Tech companies: channel partnerships, 221–25; health care ventures of,
223–24; marketplaces, 223; philosophy
of "self-serve," 222

Biofourmis, 32

Biovitals Analytics Engine, 32–33

BioXcel Therapeutics, 266

blood pressure control study, 238–39

Blue Note Therapeutics, 84–85

Blue Ocean Strategy, 12, 69

BlueStar®, 24–28, 241

BlueStar's Insulin Adjustment Program
(IAP), 26, 87–88

Booty, Edward, 216

brain rehabilitation therapy, 83

Breazeal, Cynthia, 263

Brocklebank, Nicholas, 122

BT Group, 218

business planning tools, 95

business-to-business (B2B) model, 73,
112n7, 197–98, 232, 241

business-to-business-to-consumer (B2B2C)
model, 197, 198, 219, 241, 247

business-to-consumer (B2C) model, 73,
112n7, 197, 198, 219, 232, 241, 247

business-to-payer model, 232

business ventures, 96, 97, 98, 99

business viability, 91, 95, 96

Buyer Utility Map, 64

buying decision process, 68–73

Cahill, Ken, 31

cancer: screening, 218; statistics, 3

capitation, 223

cardiovascular diseases, 3, 33

care delivery: variability of, 113–15

Centers for Medicare & Medicaid
Services, 214

chain of buyers, 69–70, 72–73

channel partnerships: with Big Tech
companies, 221–25; with employers,
206–10; with insurance companies,
210–13; key factors of, 227; with
medical device companies, 202–3;
models of, 229; as path to DTx
distribution and commercialization,
10–11, 193, 194, 197, 198–200, 242–43,
254–55; with pharmaceutical companies,

200–202, 204–5, 226, 254–55; with
pharmaceutical distributors, 203–4;
recommendations for, 228–29; with
telecommunications companies,
217–21, 226; with teleX organizations,
214–17

chatbots, 261

ChatGPT, 262

checklists, 39

China Mobile, 218

chloroquine, 133

Christensen, Clayton M., 57

chronic diseases, 3, 4, 104–5, 209

chronic obstructive pulmonary disease
(COPD), 202

Cigna, 213, 244

Cincinnati Children's Hospital, 235

Click Therapeutics, 27

click-through rates (CTRs), 106, 107, 108

clinical endpoints, 131

clinical evidence, 29, 256

clinical needs, 10, 41, 77, 88–89

clinical trials: data collection, 146–47,
151; data storage and sharing, 147;
design and execution of, 131, 151;
enrollment practices, 30–31

ClinicalTrials.gov, 129

clinicaltrialsregister.eu, 129

Clinical Trials Transformation Initiative
(CTTI), 133, 145, 148

clinical validation, 113, 130, 136–38, 150,
151

cloud platforms, 218

cognitive behavioral stress management
(CBSM), 85

cognitive behavioral therapy (CBT), 84,
85, 178

cognitive bias, 103

compensatory behaviors, 61

concept tests, 109

Conference on Computer and Communications Security, 125

Conference on Neural Information
Processing Systems, 125

Connected Clinical Trials (CCT), 146

CONSORT 2010 Statement, 142

contract research organizations (CROs),
130

digital therapeutics (DTx) (*cont.*)
related to, 111n4; capabilities of, 34–35; checklists for, 40; clinical evidence of effectiveness of, 28–29, 136; continuous evolution of, 165–66, 167; cultural setting and, 135–36; data privacy and, 124; definition of, 3, 22–24, 266; demand-driven *vs.* supply-driven, 64; development of, 135, 226; *vs.* digital health solutions, 21, 24, 32; distribution strategies for, 194, 197–98, 227; economic value of, 193–94; effectiveness of, 154; emotional proposition, 67; evidence-based framework, 98, 270, 272; evolution of, 250–51, 254; examples of, 27–28; feedback of users, 252; foundational principles of, 23; global market, 123, 192–93; guidelines for, 137–38; identification of pain points, 74; impact on clinical and financial outcomes, 87; intellectual property and, 98–99; JTBD framework, 58–60; local context, 236; measures of performance of, 137; outcomes of, 27–28; patient-focused nature of, 35, 88, 256; potential of, xi, 4–5, 10, 255–56; as prescription-based products, 35, 254; private- and public-sector financing of, 247; problem-solving capabilities, 39–40; proliferation of, 192–93; public payers, 232–36; real-world evidence (RWE) of effectiveness of, 30, 31, 234–35, 245, 255; regulation of, 137, 138, 148, 149–50, 194, 232–33, 234, 245; regulatory approval, 31–35, 130, 148, 251; risk-based classification of, 148–49; roadmap to scalability of, 9; role of qualitative research in development of, 136; stakeholder ecosystem, 46, 47, 55; standard of care *vs.*, 133–35; strategic focus areas, 104; subcategories of, 26; test-and-learn approach, 102–4, 110, 111; test for efficacy, 138; users of, 101, 111n1, 112n7, 156–57; validation of, 10, 128, 135–36, 137, 150–51; value proposition, 104, 134; *vs.* wellness apps, 10; work in practice, 24. *See also* implementation of DTx solutions

Digital Therapeutics Alliance (DTA), 22, 266
dilution of control, 96, 99n7
direct-to-consumer distribution model, 205
diseases: statistics, 82; top 10 causes of death, 24, 82, 90n13
disruptive technologies, 224
distribution services, 203–4, 205
DKSH, 203
DNA sequencing, 7
Dose Adjustment for Normal Eating program, 52
drugs: dosing methods, 140, 141; *vs.* supplements, 31–32
Drugstore.com, 223
DTx commercialization: challenges of, 226; channel partnerships as path to, 10–11, 193, 194, 197, 198–99, 242–43, 254–55; common blind spots, 193–94; regulatory requirements, 129–30; studies of, 195n8
DTx pricing: considerations for selecting, 240–41, 247; DTx as a service approach, 242; franchise model, 242; geographical considerations for, 242; hybrid models, 247; importance of real-world evidence, 234–35, 245–46; one-off payment model, 240; private payers, 236–37; public payers, 233–36; return-on-investment-based model, 235, 237, 246; revenue sharing with distribution channels, 242; subscription model, 240, 246; users' willingness to pay and, 237–39; value-based model, 231, 235, 237, 243–46
Dutch health care system, 79–80

economic evaluation studies, 129
effectiveness *vs.* efficacy, 137
e-health, 154–55, 161n4, 169
eHealth Stakeholder Group, 34
electronic health records (EHRs), 6, 8, 165
emotions, 64
Employee Health Association, 207
employers: benefits schemes, 236; channel partnerships, 206–10; DTx innovations and, 207–8, 209; as health

milestone planning chart, 95
mindline.sg, 234
mobile health tools, 2, 24, 142, 169
multiarm trials, 134
multimorbidity, 79–80
multiple sclerosis (MS), 78, 87
multivariate tests, 110
musculoskeletal disorders, 98
music therapy, 77–78

Naluri, 202, 246
National Cancer Screening Registry
    (Australia), 218
National Health Service (NHS) (UK), 218
National Institute for Health and Care
    Excellence (NICE), 137
National University Health System
    (NUHS) (Singapore), 180
net monetary benefit (NMB), positive, 178
Neupro, 133
neural network, 265
neurological diseases, 82–83, 193
neurologic music therapy, 77
Ngiam, Kee Yuan, 13–14, 119, 163
N-of-1 (personalized) clinical trials:
    CONSORT extension for, 142–43;
    development of, 86; digital therapeu-
    tics for, 88, 151; implementation prob-
    lems, 29; improvements in data analyt-
    ics, 139–40; intervention sequence,
    139; IRB review process, 142; as path-
    way toward individualized treatments,
    143; patient-centric design of, 87, 139;
    vs. randomized clinical trials (RCTs), 30
nonadoption, abandonment, spread,
    scale-up, and sustainability (NASSS)
    framework, 170
North East London National Health
    System Foundation Trust (UK), 235
Novartis, 244
nurses, 81

Omada digital DPP program, 213
Omada Health, 84
Oon, Matt, 15, 89, 270, 272, 273–74
OpenMined, 122, 125
operational pivots, 109
ophthalmologists, 81

Organisation for Economic Co-operation
    and Development, 206, 238
Osman-Rani, Azran, 74
Otsuka Pharmaceutical, 193, 195n8, 200,
    201, 204
outcomes-based deals, 244
outer setting, 155
overhead costs, 93

pain management, 83–84
pain points, 64, 66, 74
painted door test, 107–8
Parkinson's disease, 77, 78, 82
PathAI, 265
Patient Centered Outcomes Research
    Institute, 182
patient-centered solutions, 157
patient-physician relationships, 177–78,
    180, 182–84, 253–54
patients: behavior mechanisms used to
    nudge, 186, 187–88; DTx potential
    for, 7, 56, 179–82, 251–52, 256; first
    consultation with a specialist, 47; peer
    support, 183–84; teleX organizations
    and, 214
PatientsLikeMe (online community), 183
Pear Therapeutics, 27, 28n7, 33, 200,
    215–16, 230n19
Penn Medicine, 186, 188
personalized medicine, 7, 86–87
Pfizer, 44, 45
pharmaceutical companies: challenges of,
    199–200; data-sharing agreements,
    201–2; drug-plus programs, 201; DTx
    partnerships, 82, 193, 200–202, 204–5,
    226, 254–55
pharmaceutical distributors, 203–4
physicians: caring for patients with
    diabetes, 50–51, 52; DTx solutions
    and, 7, 56, 174, 175–76
Pichai, Sundar, 123
pilot studies, 113–14
Ping An Good Doctor, 215, 222
plan-do-study-act (PDSA) method, 168,
    169
prescription medications, 238
price elasticity analysis, 239
Privacy Project, The, 123

Teladoc, 94, 215, 217
telcos (telecommunications companies): B2C and B2B2C business models, 219; data privacy and security regulations, 218; health care services, 218, 220; partnerships, 217–21, 226; reputational risk, 219; subscription-based models, 219; technical capacities, 218
telehealth (teleX): basic models, 214; cross-selling potential, 217; delivery of health care, 214–15; DTx partnerships, 214–17; expansion of, 7, 214–15; laws and policies, 214; patient-provider interaction, 214; privacy concerns, 214; user satisfaction, 215
Telstra, 218
"test and learn" culture, 101, 102–3, 110
theory of mind AI, 263
therapy nonadherence, 53–54
Time BioVentures, vii
tobacco users: engagement with digital tools, 183
total addressable market (TAM), 91, 92, 99n1
transaction tests, 109
traumatic brain injury, 82
treatment: dosing adjustments, 86; personalized approaches, 85–86; side effects, 86; use of artificial intelligence, 86, 140–41

UCB Biopharma, 133
unified theory of acceptance, 155
United Kingdom: DTx regulations, 33–34

United States: diabetes therapy nonadherence, 53; DTx regulations, 34; health care expenditures, 244
UpScript Health, 215–16
Us2.ai medtech company, 7
usability: as factor affecting new technology, 156–57
utility levers, 64, 65, 66, 68

value: concept of, 193–94
value-added services (VAS), 210, 211–12
value-based contracting schemes, 247
value-based health care: development of, 231, 232; DTx pricing and, 243; patients' perspective on, 232, 243–44; providers' perspective on, 232–33
value of investment (VOI): vs. return on investment (ROI), 207
video games, 134
Voluntis, 28

waitlist-based control groups, 134, 135
Wallach, D. A., vii
weak AI, 259, 260–61
Welldoc Inc., 24, 28, 241
wellness and support, 21, 22
wellness apps, 10
Wellthy Therapeutics, 202
World Health Organization, 39, 53
Wysa, 235

Yeo, Geck Hong, 89, 270, 272–73, 274
Yeoh, Ester, 11–12, 43, 47, 51, 52, 55

Zuellig Pharma, 203–4

About the Authors

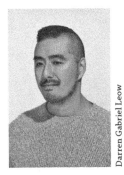

Darren Gabriel Leow

Dean Ho
Provost's Chair Professor, Director of the Institute for Digital Medicine (WisDM), Director of the N.1 Institute for Health, and Head of the Department of Biomedical Engineering at the National University of Singapore

Dean Ho and collaborators successfully developed and validated CURATE. AI, a powerful artificial intelligence platform that personalizes human treatment for a broad spectrum of indications ranging from oncology to digital therapeutics and infectious diseases, among others.

Ho is an elected fellow of the National Academy of Inventors. He is also a fellow of the American Association for the Advancement of Science, the American Institute for Medical and Biological Engineering, and the Royal Society of Chemistry. He was named to the Healthcare Information and Management Systems Society's Future50 Class of 2021 for his internationally recognized contributions to digital health and is a subgroup lead in the World Health Organization's Working Group on Regulatory Considerations for AI in Health.

Ho has appeared on the National Geographic Channel's *Known Universe* and Channel News Asia's *The Hidden Layer: Healthcare Trailblazers*. His discoveries have been featured on CNN and NPR and in the *Economist*, *Forbes*, and the *Washington Post*, among other international news outlets. He has also served as the president of the board of directors of the Society for Laboratory Automation and Screening, a global drug development organization comprised of senior executives from the pharmaceutical and medical device sectors as well as academic visionaries.

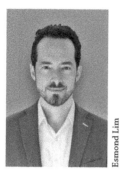

Yoann Sapanel

Head of Health Innovation, the Institute for Digital Medicine (WisDM) at the Yong Loo Lin School of Medicine, National University of Singapore

Yoann Sapanel, passionate about bridging the efficacy-effectiveness gap for digital therapeutics, is an expert in medical technology development driven by payer perspectives.

At WisDM, Sapanel aims to foster and accelerate cross-industry, public–private collaborations to validate, implement, and scale pioneering pharmacological and digital interventional technologies into the clinic. As a member of the Singapore Health District initiative, he designs, evaluates, and drives the implementation of technological solutions within the community to support resident's health through life stages.

Prior to that, Sapanel was the head of Health Partnerships at MetLife, focusing on the development of new products and services grounded in technology and data for cancer, dementia, and cardiovascular diseases. In that role, he led the implementation of the world's first mobile, clinically valid, neurocognitive assessment test and mobile app for improving brain health in Japan.

Earlier, Sapanel led the Asia Pacific Center of Excellence for Business Model Innovation at Medtronic, where he designed, executed, and scaled the company's first specialized clinic for the management of heart failure patients. As program director for Medtronic Asia's Value-Based Health Care Council, he was instrumental in advancing the adoption of outcome-based models to ensure better patients outcomes, reduce costs, and deliver value across the region.

As consultant at Blue Ocean Strategy and PwC, Sapanel also conducted strategy formulation projects with leading pharmaceutical companies.

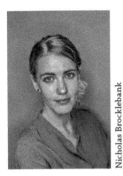

Nicholas Brocklebank

Agata Blasiak
Research Assistant Professor and Head of Digital Health Innovation at the Institute for Digital Medicine (WisDM) and the N.1 Institute for Health at the National University Singapore

Agata Blasiak is a developer and implementer of digital health technologies. She has codeveloped several digital platforms for decentralized health care that are in the process of being clinically validated and has collaborated with leading health startup innovators. Beyond technical development, Blasiak's research areas of interest are behavioral and societal aspects of digital health solutions as catalysts for the holistic translation of inventions into innovations that have a positive impact on patients.

At WisDM and N.1, Blasiak's work has focused on leveraging CURATE.AI for personalized dosing in oncology. Her work has also harnessed IDentif. AI—an AI platform for optimizing combination therapies for infectious diseases—to rapidly pinpoint actionable drug combinations against SARS-CoV-2 and other infectious diseases. She has received multiple awards for her work, including *MIT Technology Review* recognition as a member of the Innovators Under 35 Asia Pacific 2021.

Before venturing into the digital health space, Blasiak was a neuroengineer researcher and focused her efforts on molecular neuroengineering and developing neuroimplants. She holds a BScEng in biotechnology from Warsaw University of Technology, Poland, and a PhD in bionano interactions from University College Dublin, Ireland.